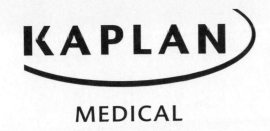

MEDICAL

USMLE®

STEP 2 CK
Lecture Notes 2018

Surgery

© 2017 by Kaplan, Inc.

Published by Kaplan Medical, a division of Kaplan, Inc.
750 Third Avenue
New York, NY 10017

10 9 8 7 6 5 4 3 2 1

Course ISBN: 978-1-5062-2822-8

Retail Kit ISBN: 978-1-5062-2088-8
This item comes as a set and should not be broken out and sold separately.

Kaplan Publishing print books are available at special quantity discounts to use for sales promotions, employee premiums, or educational purposes. For more information or to purchase books, please call the Simon & Schuster special sales department at 866-506-1949.

Editors

Carlos Pestana, M.D., Ph.D.
Emeritus Professor of Surgery
University of Texas Medical School at San Antonio
San Antonio, TX

Adil Farooqui, M.D., F.R.C.S.
Clinical Assistant Professor of Surgery
Keck School of Medicine, University of Southern California
Kaiser Permanente, West Los Angeles Medical Center
Los Angeles, CA

Mark Nolan Hill, M.D., F.A.C.S.
Professor of Surgery
Chicago Medical School
Chicago, IL

Contributor

Ted A. James, M.D., M.S., F.A.C.S.
Chief, Breast Surgical Oncology
Vice Chair, Academic Affairs
Department of Surgery
Beth Israel Deaconess Medical Center
Harvard Medical School
Boston, MA

The editors wish to also acknowledge **Gary Schwartz**, M.D., Baylor University Medical Center.

We want to hear what you think. What do you like or not like about the Notes? Please email us at **medfeedback@kaplan.com**.

Table of Contents

Part I. Surgery

Part II. Surgical Vignettes

Additional resources available at
www.kaptest.com/usmlebookresources

PART I

Surgery

Trauma 1

Learning Objectives

❑ List the ABCs of evaluating a trauma patient

❑ Demonstrate a head-to-toe review of a trauma patient

❑ Provide basic information about treatment of burns, bites, and stings

PRIMARY SURVEY: THE ABCs

Airway

The first step in the evaluation of trauma is airway assessment and protection.

- An airway is considered protected if the patient is conscious and speaking in a normal tone of voice.
- An airway is considered unprotected if there is an expanding hematoma or subcutaneous emphysema in the neck, noisy or "gurgly" breathing, or a Glasgow Coma Scale <8.

An airway should be secured before the situation becomes critical. **In the field,** an airway can be secured by intubation or cricothyroidotomy. This is called a "definitive airway." **In the emergency department**, it is best done by rapid sequence induction and orotracheal intubation, with monitoring of pulse oximetry. In the presence of a cervical spine injury, orotracheal intubation can still be done as long as the head is secured and in-line stabilization is maintained during the procedure. Another option in that setting is nasotracheal intubation over a fiberoptic bronchoscope. If severe maxillofacial injuries preclude the use of intubation or intubation is unsuccessful, cricothyroidotomy may become necessary.

In the pediatric patient population (age <12), tracheostomy is preferred over cricothyroidotomy due to the high risk of airway stenosis, as the cricoid is much smaller than in the adult.

Breathing

Breath sounds indicate **satisfactory ventilation**; an absence or decrease of breath sounds may indicate a pneumothorax and/or hemothorax and necessitate chest tube placement. **Pulse oximetry** indicates **satisfactory oxygenation**; hypoxia may be secondary to airway compromise, pulmonary contusion, or neurological injury impairing respiratory drive and necessitate intubation. Measurement of CO_2 (capnography) is also very useful.

Circulation

Clinical signs of shock include the following:

- Low BP (<90 mm Hg systolic)
- Tachycardia (heart rate >100 bpm)
- Low urinary output (<0.5 ml/kg/h)

Patients in shock will be pale, cold, shivering, sweating, thirsty, and apprehensive.

In the trauma setting, shock is either hypovolemic (secondary to hemorrhage and the most common scenario) or cardiogenic (secondary to pericardial tamponade or tension pneumothorax due to chest trauma).

Hemorrhagic shock tends to cause collapsed neck veins due to low central venous pressure (CVP), while cardiogenic shock tends to cause elevated CVP with jugular venous distention. Both processes may occur simultaneously.

In pericardial tamponade, there is typically no respiratory distress, while in tension pneumothorax there is significant dyspnea, loss of unilateral breath sounds, and tracheal deviation.

Treatment of hemorrhagic shock includes volume resuscitation and control of bleeding, in the OR or ED depending on the injury and available resources. Volume resuscitation is initially with 2L of Lactated Ringer's solution unless blood products are immediately available.

In the setting of trauma, transfusion of blood products should be in a 1:1:1 ratio between packed RBCs, fresh frozen plasma, and platelets. Resuscitation should be continued until BP and heart rate normalize and urine output reaches 0.5–1.0 ml/kg/hr. In the setting of uncontrolled hemorrhage, permissive hypotension is recommended to prevent further blood loss while awaiting definitive surgical repair, but a mean arterial pressure >60 mm Hg should be maintained to ensure adequate cerebral perfusion.

The preferred route of fluid resuscitation in the trauma setting is 2 large bore peripheral IV lines, 16-gauge or greater. If this cannot be obtained, percutaneous subclavian or femoral vein catheters should be inserted; an acceptable alternative is a saphenous vein cut-down. In children age <6, intraosseus cannulation of the proximal tibia or femur is the alternate route.

Pericardial tamponade is generally a clinical diagnosis and can be confirmed with U/S. Management requires evacuation of the pericardial space by pericardiocentesis, subxiphoid pericardial window, or thoracotomy. Fluid and blood administration while evacuation is being set up is helpful to maintain an adequate cardiac output..

Tension pneumothorax is a clinical diagnosis based on physical exam. Management requires immediate decompression of the pleural space, initially with a large-bore needle which converts the tension to a simple pneumothorax and followed by chest tube placement.

In the non-trauma setting, shock can also be hypovolemic because of massive fluid loss such as bleeding, burns, peritonitis, pancreatitis, or massive diarrhea. The clinical picture is similar to trauma, with hypotension, tachycardia, and oliguria with a low CVP. Stop the bleeding and replace the blood volume.

Intrinsic cardiogenic shock is caused by myocardial damage (e.g. myocardial infarction or fulminant myocarditis). The clinical picture is hypotension, tachycardia, and oliguria with a high CVP (presenting as distended neck veins). Treat with pharmacologic circulatory support. Differential diagnosis is essential, because additional fluid and blood administration in this setting could be lethal, as the failing heart becomes easily overloaded.

Vasomotor shock (from anaphylaxis, high spinal anesthesia, or spinal cord transection) causes circulatory collapse. Patients are flushed, "pink and warm" with a low CVP. Treatment with phenylephrine and fluids is aimed at filling dilated veins and restoring peripheral resistance.

SECONDARY SURVEY

After the ABC's have been evaluated and any immediate life-threatening emergencies addressed, trauma evaluation continues with the secondary survey which is composed of a complete physical exam to evaluate for occult injuries followed by chest x-ray and pelvic x-ray. The secondary survey may be augmented with further imaging studies depending on the mechanism of injury and findings on examination. Any change that occurs requires complete re-evaluation.

A REVIEW FROM HEAD TO TOE

Head Trauma

- Penetrating head trauma as a rule requires surgical intervention and repair of the damage.
- Linear skull fractures are left alone if they are closed (no overlying wound).
- Open fractures require wound closure. If comminuted or depressed, treat in the OR.
- Anyone with head trauma who has become unconscious gets a CT scan to look for intracranial hematomas. If negative and neurologically intact, they can go home if the family will awaken them frequently during the next 24 hours to make sure they are not going into coma.

Signs of a fracture affecting the base of the skull include raccoon eyes, rhinorrhea, otorrhea or ecchymosis behind the ear (Battle's sign). CT scan of the head is required to rule out intracranial bleeding and should be extended to include the neck to evaluate for a cervical spinal injury. Expectant management is the rule and antibiotics are not usually indicated.

Neurologic damage from trauma can be caused by 3 components:

- Initial blow
- Subsequent development of a hematoma that displaces the midline structures
- Later development of increased intracranial pressure (ICP) due to cerebral edema

There is no treatment for the first (other than prevention), surgery can relieve the second, and medical measures can prevent or minimize the third.

Acute epidural hematoma occurs with modest trauma to the side of the head, and has a classic sequence of trauma, unconsciousness, a lucid interval (a completely asymptomatic patient who returns to his previous activity), gradual lapsing into coma again, fixed dilated pupil (90% of the time on the side of the hematoma), and contralateral hemiparesis with decerebrate posturing. CT scan shows a biconvex, lens-shaped hematoma. Emergency craniotomy produces a dramatic cure. Because every patient who has been unconscious gets a CT scan, the full-blown picture with the fixed pupil and contralateral hemiparesis is seldom seen.

Acute subdural hematoma has the same sequence, but the force of the trauma is typically much larger and the patient is usually much sicker (not fully awake and asymptomatic at any point), due to more severe neurologic damage. CT scan will show semilunar, crescent-shaped hematoma. If midline structures are deviated, craniotomy will help, but prognosis is bad. If there is no deviation, therapy is centered on preventing further damage from subsequent increased ICP.

Invasive ICP monitoring, head elevation, modest hyperventilation, avoidance of fluid over-load, and diuretics such as mannitol or furosemide can decrease ICP. However, do not diurese to the point of lowering systemic arterial pressure, as **cerebral perfusion pressure = mean arterial pressure minus intracranial pressure**. Hyperventilation is recommended when there are signs of herniation, and the goal is PCO2 35 mm Hg. Sedation is used to decrease brain activity and oxygen demand. Moderate hypothermia is currently recommended to further reduce cerebral oxygen demand.

Diffuse axonal injury occurs in more severe trauma. CT scan shows diffuse blurring of the gray-white matter interface and multiple small punctate hemorrhages. Without hematoma there is no role for surgery. Therapy is directed at preventing further damage from increased ICP.

Chronic subdural hematoma occurs in the very old or in severe alcoholics. A shrunken brain is rattled around the head by minor trauma, tearing venous sinuses. Over several days or weeks, mental function deteriorates as hematoma forms. CT scan is diagnostic, and surgical evacuation provides a dramatic cure.

Hypovolemic shock cannot happen from intracranial bleeding: there isn't enough space inside the head for the amount of blood loss needed to produce shock. Look for another source.

Neck Trauma

For the purpose of evaluating penetrating neck trauma, the neck has been divided into 3 zones.
- From caudad to cephalad, **zone 1** extends from the clavicles to the cricoid cartilage
- **Zone 2** from the cricoic cartilage to the angle of the mandible
- **Zone 3** from the angle of the mandible to the base of the skull

Penetrating trauma to the neck mandates surgical exploration in all cases where there is an expanding hematoma, deteriorating vital signs, or signs of esophageal or tracheal injury such as coughing or spitting up blood.
- For injuries to zone 1, evaluate with angiography, esophagogram (water-soluble, fol-lowed by barium if negative), esophagoscopy, and bronchoscopy to help decide if sur-gical exploration is indicated and to determine the ideal surgical approach.
- Historically, all penetrating injuries to zone 2 mandated surgical exploration, with a recent trend toward selective exploration based on physical exam.
  - If the patient is stable with low index of suspicion of a significant injury, use the above diagnostic modalities to evaluate the situation and potentially avoid unneces-sary surgical exploration.
  - If the patient's condition changes, however, urgent surgical exploration is indicated.
- For injuries to zone 3, evaluate with angiography for vascular injury.

In all patients with severe blunt trauma to the neck, the integrity of the cervical spine has to be ascertained. Unconscious patients and conscious patients with midline tenderness to pal-pation should be evaluated initially with CT scan, and potentially followed with MRI depend-ing on findings. Conscious patients with no symptoms (are not intoxicated, have not used drugs, or have no 'distracting' injury) can be clinically evaluated for a cervical spinal injury; however if CT scan of the head is being obtained, it is generally accepted to extend the study to include the cervical spine.

Spinal Cord Injury

Complete transection is unlikely to be on the exam because it is too easy: nothing works, sensory, or motor, below the level of the injury.

Hemisection (Brown-Sequard) is typically caused by a clean-cut injury such as a knife blade, and results in ipsilateral paralysis and loss of proprioception and contralateral loss of pain perception caudal to the level of the injury.

Anterior cord syndrome is typically seen in burst fractures of the vertebral bodies. There is loss of motor function and loss of pain and temperature sensation on both sides caudal to the injury, with preservation of vibratory and positional sense.

Central cord syndrome occurs in the elderly with forced hyperextension of the neck, such as a rear-end collision. There is paralysis and burning pain in the upper extremities, with preservation of most functions in the lower extremities.

Management necessitates precise diagnosis of a cord injury, best done with MRI. There is some evidence that high-dose corticosteroids immediately after the injury may help, but that concept is still controversial. Further surgical management is too specialized for the exam.

Chest Trauma

Rib fractures can be deadly in the elderly, because pain impairs respiratory effort, which leads to hypoventilation, atelectasis, and ultimately, pneumonia. To avoid this cycle, treat pain from rib fractures with a local nerve block or epidural catheter, in addition to oral and IV analgesics.

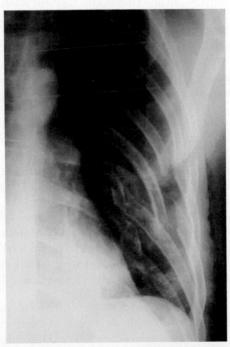

Figure I-1-1. X-ray of Multiple Rib Fractures due to Trauma

Simple pneumothorax results from penetrating trauma such as a weapon or the jagged edge of a fractured rib. There is typically moderate shortness of breath with absence of unilateral breath sounds and hyperresonance to percussion. Diagnosis is confirmed with chest x-ray, and management consists of chest tube placement.

Hemothorax happens the same way but the affected side will be dull to percussion due to blood accumulation in the pleural space. The blood can originate directly from the lung parenchyma or from the chest wall, such as an intercostal artery. Diagnosis is confirmed with chest x-ray. Chest tube placement is necessary to enable evacuation of the accumulated blood to prevent late development of a fibrothorax or empyema, but surgery to stop the bleeding is sometimes required. If the lung is the source of bleeding, it usually stops spontaneously as it is a low pressure system.

In some cases where a systemic vessel such as an intercostal artery is the source of bleeding, thoracotomy is needed to stop the hemorrhage. Indications for thoracotomy include:

- Evacuation of >1,500 mL when the chest tube is inserted
- Collecting drainage of >1 L of blood over 4 hours, i.e., 250 mL/hr

Severe blunt trauma to the chest may cause obvious injuries such as rib fractures with a flail chest or sucking chest wound, as well as less apparent injuries such as pulmonary contusion, blunt cardiac injury, diaphragmatic injury, and aortic injury.

Sucking chest wounds are obvious from physical exam, as there is a flap that sucks air with inspiration and closes during expiration. Untreated, it will lead to a deadly tension pneumothorax. Initial management is with a partially occlusive dressing secured on 3 sides, with one open side acting as a one-way valve. This allows air to escape but not to enter the pleural cavity (to prevent iatrogenic tension pneumothorax and multiple fractures within each rib).

Flail chest occurs with multiple rib fractures that allow a segment of the chest wall to cave in during inspiration and bulge out during expiration (paradoxical breathing). The real problem is the underlying pulmonary contusion. A contused lung is very sensitive to fluid overload, thus treatment includes fluid restriction and pain management. Pulmonary dysfunction may develop, thus serial chest x-rays and arterial blood gases have to be monitored.

Pulmonary contusion can show up right away after chest trauma with "white-out" of the affected lung(s) or can be delayed up to 48 hours. If a respirator is needed, bilateral chest tubes should be considered to prevent a tension pneumothorax from developing as the multiple broken ribs may have punctured the lung. Significant force is necessary to result in a flail chest, so traumatic dissection or transection of the aorta should be evaluated for using a CT angiogram. Finally, ARDS may develop in this scenario.

Blunt cardiac injury should be suspected with the presence of sternal fractures. ECG monitoring will detect any abnormalities. Although serum troponin level was historically obtained, elevations do not generally change management and are therefore not indicated, as treatment is focused on the complications of the injury such as arrhythmias.

Traumatic rupture of the diaphragm shows up with the bowel in the chest (by physical exam and x-rays), almost always on the left side (the liver protects the right hemidiaphragm). All suspicious cases should be evaluated with laparoscopy. Surgical repair is typically done from the abdomen.

Traumatic rupture of the aorta is the ultimate "hidden injury." It most commonly occurs at the junction of the arch and the descending aorta where the relatively mobile aorta is tethered by the ligamentum arteriosum. Such an injury requires a significant deceleration injury and is totally asymptomatic until the hematoma contained by the adventitia ruptures resulting in rapid death. Suspicion should be triggered by one of the following:

- Mechanism of injury
- Widened mediastinum on chest x-ray
- Presence of atypical fractures such as the first rib, scapula, or sternum, which requires great force to fracture

Diagnosis is made with CT angiogram. Surgical repair is indicated once the patient has been stabilized and more immediate live-threatening injuries have been managed. This can be done in an open or endovascular fashion.

Traumatic rupture of the trachea or major bronchus is suggested by developing subcutaneous emphysema in the upper chest and lower neck, or by a large "air leak" from a chest tube. Chest x-ray and CT scan confirm the presence of air outside the bronchopulmonary tree, and fiberoptic bronchoscopy is necessary to identify the injury and allow intubation past the injury to secure an airway. Surgical repair is indicated.

Differential diagnosis of **subcutaneous emphysema** also includes rupture of the esophagus and tension pneumothorax.

Air embolism should be suspected when sudden death occurs in a chest trauma patient who is intubated and on a respirator. It also can occur when the subclavian vein is opened to the air (e.g. supraclavicular node biopsies, central venous line placement or lines that become disconnected), also leading to sudden cardiovascular collapse and cardiac arrest. Immediate management includes cardiac massage, with the patient positioned in Trendelenburg with the left side down. Prevention includes the Trendelenburg position when the great veins at the base of the neck are to be accessed.

Fat embolism may also produce respiratory distress in a trauma patient who may not have necessarily suffered chest trauma. The typical setting is the following:

- Patient with multiple traumatic injuries (including several long bone fractures) develops petechial rashes in the axillae and neck; fever, tachycardia, and low platelet count
- At some point patient shows a full-blown picture of respiratory distress, with hypoxemia and bilateral patchy infiltrates on chest x-ray

The mainstay of therapy is respiratory support, and therefore precise diagnosis is not needed and rarely confirmed. Other therapies for this syndrome including heparin, steroids, alcohol, or low-molecular-weight dextran have been discredited.

Abdominal Trauma

For the sake of evaluation and management, abdominal trauma is divided into penetrating and blunt trauma based on the mechanism of injury. **Penetrating trauma** is further differentiated into gunshot wounds and stab wounds as the pattern of injury based on mechanism is quite different.

- Gunshot wounds to the abdomen require exploratory laparotomy for evaluation and possible repair of intra-abdominal injuries, not to "remove the bullet." Any entrance or exit wound below the level of the nipple line is considered to involve the abdomen.
- Stab wounds allow a more individualized approach. If it is clear that penetration has occurred, e.g. protruding viscera, exploratory laparotomy is mandatory.
- The same is true if hemodynamic instability or signs of peritoneal irritation develop.

In the absence of the conditions above, local wound exploration may be performed in the ED to assess whether or not the anterior rectus fascia has been penetrated.

- If the fascia is not violated, the intra-abdominal cavity likely has not been penetrated and no further intervention is necessary.
- If the fascia has been violated, surgical exploration is indicated to evaluate for bowel or vascular injury, even in the setting of hemodynamic stability and lack of peritoneal findings on physical examination. If there is any question, perform CT.

Blunt trauma to the abdomen with obvious signs of internal injury requires emergent surgical evaluation via exploratory laparotomy. Signs of internal injury include abdominal distention and significant abdominal pain with guarding or rigidity on physical examination consistent with peritonitis. The occurrence of blunt trauma even without obvious signs of internal injury requires further evaluation because internal hemorrhage or bowel injury can be slow and therefore present in a delayed fashion.

Signs of internal bleeding include a drop in BP, a fast and/or thready pulse, a low CVP, and low urinary output. Patients tend to be cold, pale, anxious, shivering, thirsty, and perspiring profusely. These signs of shock occur when 25–30% of blood volume is acutely lost, ~1,500 ml in the average-size adult. There are few places in the body that this volume of blood can be lost without being obvious on physical or radiographic exam.

- The head is too small without causing a lethal degree of intracranial pressure.
- The neck could contain a significant amount of blood, but such a hematoma would be obvious on physical exam.
- The pericardial sac cannot contain a significant amount of blood loss without resulting in pericardial tamponade and rapid clinical deterioration.
- The pleural cavities could easily accommodate several liters of blood, with relatively few local symptoms, but that significant a hemothorax would be obvious on chest x-ray, which is routinely performed in the secondary survey of a trauma patient.
- The arms and legs would also be obviously deformed by a large hematoma if present.

That leaves the abdomen, retroperitoneum, thighs (secondary to a femur fracture), and pelvis as the only places where a volume of blood significant enough to cause shock could "hide" in a blunt trauma patient that has become unstable. The femurs and pelvis are always checked for fractures in the initial survey of the trauma patient by physical exam and pelvic x-ray. So a patient who has experienced blunt trauma who has become hemodynamically unstable with normal chest and pelvic x-rays likely has intra-abdominal bleeding.

Diagnosis can be quickly utilizing the "FAST" exam: **F**ocused **A**bdominal **S**onography for **T**rauma. Bedside U/S evaluates the perihepatic space, perisplenic space, pelvis, and pericardium for free fluid. Fluid is not typically present in these locations, so if there is a clinical suspicion such as hypotension following blunt trauma, consider an internal injury.

- An unstable patient with these findings should be taken to the OR for immediate surgical exploration.
- A stable patient in whom the diagnosis is less definite should be taken for a more definitive study, i.e., CT scan. CT will show the presence of intra-abdominal fluid and can accurately delineate the source, typically the liver or spleen.

Additionally, grading scores exist for the extent of injury to these solid organs, with specific guidelines as to when a surgical intervention is indicated versus observation. The details of these guidelines are outside the scope of the exam. Generally speaking, a patient with intra-abdominal bleeding injury from the liver or spleen can be observed as long as they are hemodynamically stable or respond to fluid and blood product administration; the moment instability is mentioned in a vignette, surgical exploration is indicated.

If surgical exploration is indicated for penetrating or blunt trauma, certain principles must be employed.

- Prolonged surgical time and ongoing bleeding can lead to the "triad of death": hypothermia, coagulopathy, and acidosis. The longer a patient is open, these component worsen and precipitate each other, resulting in a vicious cycle ultimately leading to death. Accordingly, the "damage control" approach has been adopted: immediate life-threatening injuries are addressed, less urgent injuries are temporized. Obviously repair of a major vascular structure with ongoing bleeding takes precedence.
    - Next comes control of contamination from injury to the GI tract. If a bowel resection is necessary, reconstruction can be delayed as only the contamination is life-threatening, not the inability to digest food.
    - If hypothermia, coagulopathy, or acidosis is setting in and injuries have been controlled, the operation is terminated and the abdomen is packed with gauze pads and closed with a temporary closure. The patient is resuscitated in the ICU, and returns to the OR at a later date when warm, not coagulopathic, and not acidotic for definitive reconstruction and abdominal closure.
- If coagulopathy does develop during surgical exploration, it is objectively treated with transfusion of RBCs, fresh frozen plasma, and platelets in equal quantities (1:1:1 ratio). This most realistically mimics the replacement of whole blood and enables not only adequate quantities of hemoglobin, but also adequate clotting factors to reverse the developing coagulopathy and enable control of hemorrhage.
- The abdominal compartment syndrome is when the pressure in the peritoneal cavity is elevated and leads to end-organ injury. This occurs when a significant amount of fluid is administered in an effort to resuscitate a patient in hypovolemic shock. Bowel edema develops, increasing intra-abdominal pressure, which is detrimental for several reasons.
    - First, the elevated pressure leads to decreased perfusion pressure to the viscera, contributing to acute kidney injury and possibly bowel and hepatic ischemia.
    - Second, the upward pressure of the viscera on the diaphragm prevents adequate expansion of the lungs and ventilation, contributing to respiratory failure.
    - Therefore, if bowel edema is observed or intra-abdominal pressure is elevated following surgical exploration, the abdomen is not closed but rather left open as described in the damage-control approach.
    - Similarly, if a patient is not surgically explored but undergoes a significant volume resuscitation and abdominal compartment syndrome develops, a decompressive laparotomy may be indicated. Incidentally, this can occur in non-trauma scenarios requiring massive fluid resuscitation, most notably severe pancreatitis.

A **ruptured spleen** is the most common source of significant intra-abdominal bleeding in blunt abdominal trauma. Often there are additional diagnostic hints, such as fractures of lower ribs on the left side. Given the limited function of the spleen in the adult, a splenic injury resulting in hemodynamic instability or requiring significant blood product transfusion is an indication for splenectomy. Post-operative immunization against encapsulated bacteria is mandatory (pneumococcus, *Haemophilus influenza* B, and meningococcus). However, lesser injuries to the spleen which can be repaired easily are attempted.

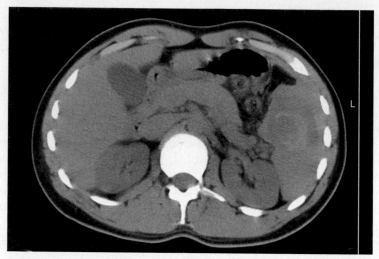

Figure I-1-2. CT Scan of Abdomen in 21-Year-Old Man demonstrating Ruptured Spleen and Hemoperitoneum

Pelvic Fracture

The pelvis is a complex ring, much like a pretzel, in that it cannot be fractured in only one location; multiple fractures are typically present. These can range from minor to life-threatening. Minor fractures with small pelvic hematomas incidentally identified on CT scan are typically monitored.

In **pelvic fracture with ongoing significant bleeding** causing hemodynamic instability, management is complex.

- The first step for an obvious pelvic fracture in an unstable patient is external pelvic wrapping for stabilization of the pelvis, which limits the potential space for ongoing blood loss.

- The next step is *not* surgical exploration but rather angiography.

  - This is because it is incredibly difficult (often impossible) to identify the source of bleeding in the pelvis where a deep cavity contains significant organs and vessels including the complex sacral venous plexus.

  - However, interventional radiologists can angiographically identify an arterial source of bleeding and potentially embolize the branch vessels and control hemorrhage.

  - If no arterial bleeding is identified, the ongoing blood loss is presumed to be venous in origin, and the internal iliac arteries are prophylactically embolized to prevent the inflow to these bleeding veins.

In any pelvic fracture, associated injuries have to be ruled out. These include injuries to the rectum (do a rectal exam and rigid proctoscopy), vagina in women (do a pelvic exam); urethra in men (do a retrograde urethrogram), and bladder (addressed in the next section).

Urologic Injury

The hallmark of urologic injury is blood in the urine of someone who has sustained penetrating or blunt abdominal trauma. Gross hematuria in that setting must be investigated with appropriate studies.

Penetrating urologic injuries as a rule are surgically explored and repaired.

- Blunt urologic injuries may affect the kidney, in which case the associated injuries tend to be lower rib fractures. If they affect the bladder or urethra, the usual associated injury is pelvic fracture.

- Urethral injuries occur almost exclusively in men. They are typically associated with a pelvic fracture, and may present with blood at the meatus.
  - Other clinical findings include a scrotal hematoma, the sensation of wanting to void but inability to do so, and a "high-riding" prostate on rectal exam (i.e., it is not palpable on rectal exam).
  - The key issue in any of these is that a **Foley catheter should not be inserted**, as it might compound an existing injury; a retrograde urethrogram should be performed instead.
    - If Foley catheter placement is attempted and resistance met, this should be a clue that a urethral injury may be present and attempt should be aborted.

- Bladder injuries can occur in either sex, are usually associated with pelvic fracture, and are diagnosed by retrograde cystogram or CT cystography.
  - The x-ray study must include post-void films to enable visualization of an extra-peritoneal leak at the base of the bladder that might be obscured by a bladder full of dye. Management is surgical repair with protection by a decompressive suprapubic cystostomy or indwelling Foley catheter.

- Renal injuries secondary to blunt trauma are usually associated with lower rib fractures. They are assessed by CT and most of the time can be managed without surgical intervention.
  - A rare but fascinating potential sequela of injuries affecting the renal pedicle is the development of an arteriovenous fistula leading to CHF. Should renal artery stenosis develop after trauma, renovascular hypertension is another potential sequela.

- Scrotal hematomas can attain alarming size, but typically do not need specific intervention unless the testicle is ruptured. The latter can be assessed with sonogram.

- Fracture of the penis (fracture of the corpora cavernosa, fracture of the tunica albuginea) occurs to an erect penis, typically as an accident during vigorous intercourse (with woman on top). There is sudden pain and development of a large penile shaft hematoma, with a normal appearing glans.
  - Frequently, the true history will be concealed by an embarrassed patient who concocts a cover story. Emergency surgical repair is required. If not done, impotence will ensue as either arteriovenous shunts or painful erections.

Injury to the Extremities

In penetrating injuries of the extremities, the main issue is whether a vascular injury has occurred or not. Anatomic location provides the first clue.

- When there are no major vessels in the vicinity of the injury, only tetanus prophylaxis and irrigation of the wound is required.
- If the penetration is near a major vessel and the patient is asymptomatic, Doppler studies or CT angiogram is performed and will guide the need for a surgical intervention.
- If there is an obvious vascular injury (absent distal pulses, expanding hematoma) surgical exploration and repair are required.

Simultaneous injuries of arteries and bone pose the challenge of the sequence of operative repair. One perspective is to stabilize the bone first, then do the delicate vascular repair which could otherwise be disrupted by the bony reduction and fixation. However during the orthopedic repair, ongoing ischemia is occurring as the arterial flow is disrupted.

A good solution, if proposed on the exam, is to place a vascular shunt, which allows temporary revascularization during the bony repair, with definitive vascular repair completed subsequently. A fasciotomy should usually be added because the prolonged ischemia could lead to a compartment syndrome.

High-velocity gunshot wounds (e.g. military or big-game hunting rifles) produce a large cone of tissue destruction that requires extensive debridements and potential amputations.

Crushing injuries of the extremities resulting in myonecrosis pose the hazard of hyperkalemia and renal failure as well as potential development of compartment syndrome. Aggressive fluid administration, osmotic diuretics, and alkalinization of the urine with sodium bicarbonate are good preventive measures for the acute kidney injury, and a fasciotomy may be required to prevent or treat compartment syndrome.

BURNS

Chemical burns require massive irrigation to remove the offending agent. Alkaline burns (Liquid Plumr, Drano) are worse than acid burns (battery acid). Irrigation must begin as soon as possible at the site where the injury occurred (tap water, shower). Do not attempt to neutralize the agent.

High-voltage electrical burns are always deeper and worse than they appear to be. Massive debridements or amputations may be required. Additional concerns include myonecrosis-induced acute kidney injury, orthopedic injuries secondary to massive muscle contractions (e.g., posterior dislocation of the shoulder, compression fractures of vertebral bodies), and late development of cataracts and demyelinization syndromes. Of course cardiac electrical integrity and function must be evaluated.

Respiratory burns (inhalation injuries) occur with flame burns in an enclosed space (a burning building, car, plane) and are chemical injuries caused by smoke inhalation. Burns around the mouth or soot inside the throat are suggestive clues. Diagnosis is confirmed with fiberoptic bronchoscopy, but the key issue is whether respiratory support is necessary, guided by serial arterial blood gases. Intubation should be initiated if there is any concern about adequacy of the airway. The routine use of tracheostomy and antibiotic/steroids therapy has been discredited, but levels of carboxyhemoglobin have to be monitored. If elevated, 100% oxygen will shorten its half-life.

Circumferential burns of the extremities can lead to tissue edema and restriction of arterial inflow, resulting in ischemia and compartment syndrome secondary to eschar. This can also occur in circumferential burns to the chest, with resultant limitations in ventilation. Escharotomies done at the bedside with no need for anesthesia will provide immediate relief.

Scalding burns in children should always raise the suspicion of child abuse, particularly if the pattern of the burn does not fit the description of the event given by the parents. A classic example is burns of both buttocks, which are typically produced by holding a small child by arms and legs, and dunking him into boiling water.

- Burns result in the loss of skin integrity and increase insensible fluid losses, leading to profound hypovolemia.
- In the first 48 hours after burn, fluid needs can be estimated by calculations that take into account the extent of the burn and provide an estimated amount of IV fluid that is needed.
- Once fluid resuscitation has been initiated, adjust based on urinary output determining the adequacy of resuscitation.
- The extent of burns in the adult is estimated by the use of the "**rule of nines**," where the head and each of the upper extremities are each assigned 9% of body surface; each lower extremity is assigned two 9% units; and trunk is assigned 4 units of 9% each.
- For purposes of most of this calculation, second- and third-degree burns are counted.

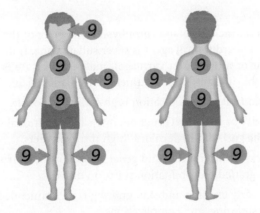

The most widely used calculation is the modified Parkland formula, in which body weight in kilograms is multiplied by the percentage of burn (as a whole number), and multiplied by 4 ml. The number obtained is the amount of Lactated Ringer's (LR) required in the first 24 hours, half of which should be infused in the first 8 hours and the other half in the next 16 hours.

Parkland Formula

> BW (kg) × % of burn (up to 50%) × 4 cc RL
>
> Infuse ½ first 8 hours, infuse ½ next 16 hours

Alternative strategy: Initiate a predetermined rate of infusion, typically 1,000 ml/h of LR for anyone whose burns >20% of body surface, and then adjust as needed to produce the desired urinary output. Fluids containing dextrose are avoided to prevent an osmotic diuresis that would render urine output unreliable as an indicator of intravascular volume status.

Estimation of fluid needs in burned babies differs from the adult in several measures.

- Babies have bigger heads and smaller legs; thus the "rule of 9s" for them assigns two 9s to the head, and both legs share a total of three 9's instead of 4.
- Third-degree burns in babies look deep bright red rather than the leathery, dry, gray appearance present in adults.
- Babies need proportionally more fluid than adults, therefore formulas and calculations in the baby use 4-6 ml/kg/%.
- A reliable predetermined rate of infusion for babies is 20 ml/kg/hour.

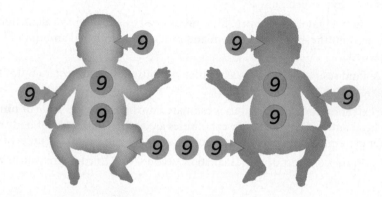

Other aspects of burn care include tetanus prophylaxis, cleaning of the burn areas, and the use of topical agents. The standard topical agent is silver sulfadiazine. If deep penetration is necessary (e.g. a thick eschar or a burn over cartilage), mafenide acetate is the choice. Burns near the eyes are covered with triple antibiotic ointment (silver sulfadiazine is irritating to the eyes).

- In the early period, all pain medication is given intravenously.
- After an initial day or two of NG suction, intensive nutritional support is provided, preferably via the gut, with high calorie/high nitrogen diets.
- After 2 or 3 weeks of wound care and general support, the burned areas that have not regenerated are grafted. Rehabilitation starts on day 1.
- When possible, early excision and skin grafting is recommended to save costs and minimize pain, suffering, and complications.

BITES AND STINGS

Tetanus prophylaxis and wound care are required for all bites. **Dog bites** are considered provoked if the dog was petted while eating or otherwise teased. No rabies prophylaxis is required, other than observation of the dog for developing signs of rabies. Because bites to the face are very close to the brain, it might be prudent to start immunization and then discontinue it if observation of the dog is reassuring.

Unprovoked dog bites or bites from wild animals raise the issue of potential rabies. If the animal is available, it can be euthanized and the brain examined for signs of rabies. Otherwise, rabies prophylaxis with immunoglobulin plus vaccine is mandatory.

Snakebites do not necessarily result in envenomation, even if the snake is poisonous (up to 30% of bitten patients are not envenomated). The most reliable signs of envenomation are severe local pain, swelling, and discoloration developing within 30 minutes of the bite. If present, draw blood for typing and crossmatch (they cannot be done later if needed), coagulation studies, and liver and renal function. Treatment is based on antivenin. The currently preferred agent for crotalids is CROFAB, of which several vials are usually needed.

Antivenin dosage relates to the size of the envenomation, not the size of the patient (children get the same dosages as adults). Surgical excision of the bite site or fasciotomy is very rarely needed. The only valid first aid is to splint the extremity during transportation. Do not make cruciate cuts, suck out venom, wrap with ice, or apply a tourniquet.

Bee stings kill many more people in the United States than snakebites because of an anaphylactic reaction. Wheezing and rash may occur, and hypotension when present is caused by vasomotor shock ("pink and warm" shock). Epinephrine is the drug of choice (0.3–0.5 ml of 1:1,000 solution). The stingers should be removed without squeezing them.

Black widow spiders are black, with a red hourglass on the belly. Bitten patients experience nausea, vomiting, and severe generalized muscle cramps. The antidote is IV calcium gluconate. Muscle relaxants also help.

Brown recluse spider bites are often not recognized at the time of the bite. In the next several days, a skin ulcer develops, with a necrotic center and a surrounding halo of erythema. Dapsone is helpful. Surgical debridement of all necrotic tissue is needed. Skin grafting may be needed subsequently.

Human bites are bacteriologically the dirtiest bite one can get. They require extensive irrigation and debridement (in the OR) and antibiotics. A classic human bite is the sharp cut over the knuckles on someone who punched someone else in the mouth and was cut by the teeth of the victim. They often show up in the ED with a cover story, but should be recognized because they need specialized orthopedic care.

Orthopedics 2

Learning Objectives

❏ Describe the diagnostic and treatment approach to common pediatric and adult orthopedic problems

❏ Answer questions about bone tumors

PEDIATRIC ORTHOPEDICS

- Congenital dysplasia of the hip runs in families, and should be ideally diagnosed right after birth. Children have uneven gluteal folds, and physical examination of the hips show that they can be easily dislocated posteriorly with a jerk and a "click," and returned to normal with a "snapping." If signs are equivocal, sonogram is diagnostic (do not order x-rays; the hip is not calcified in the newborn). Treatment is abduction splinting with a Pavlik harness for ~6 months.

- Hip pathology in older children may present as hip or knee pain. **Legg-Calve-Perthes** disease is avascular necrosis of the capital femoral epiphysis and occurs around age 6, with insidious development of limping, decreased hip motion, and hip or knee pain. Patients walk with an antalgic gait and passive motion of the hip is guarded. Diagnosis is confirmed by AP and lateral hip x-rays. Treatment is controversial, usually containing the femoral head within the acetabulum by casting and crutches.

- **Slipped capital femoral epiphysis (SCFE)** is an orthopedic emergency.
  - The typical patient is a chubby (or lanky) boy around age 13 who complains of groin or knee pain, and who ambulates with a limp.
  - When sitting with the legs dangling, the sole of the foot on the affected side points toward the other foot.
  - On physical exam there is limited hip motion, and as the hip is flexed the thigh goes into external rotation and cannot be rotated internally.
  - X-rays are diagnostic, and surgical treatment pins the femoral head back in place.

- A **septic hip** is an orthopedic emergency.
  - It is seen in toddlers who have had a febrile illness, and then refuse to move the hip. They hold the leg with the hip flexed, in slight abduction and external rotation, and do not let anybody move it passively.
  - White blood cell count and erythrocyte sedimentation rate are elevated.
  - Diagnosis is made by aspiration of the hip under general anesthesia, and further open drainage is performed if pus is obtained.

- **Acute hematogenous osteomyelitis** is seen in small children who have had a febrile illness and presents as severe localized pain in a bone with no history of trauma to that bone. X-rays will not show anything for several weeks. MRI reveals prompt diagnosis. Treatment is IV antibiotics.
- **Genu varum (bow-legs)** is normal up to age 3; no treatment is needed. Persistent varus age >3 is most commonly Blount disease, a disturbance of the medial proximal tibial growth plate, for which surgery is corrective.
- **Genu valgus (knock-knee)** is normal between ages 4–8; no treatment is needed.
- **Osgood-Schlatter disease (osteochondrosis of the tibial tubercle)** is seen in teenagers with persistent pain right over the tibial tubercle, which is aggravated by contraction of the quadriceps. Physical exam shows localized pain right over the tibial tubercle in the absence of knee swelling. Treatment is initially with rest, ice, compression, and elevation. If conservative management fails, treatment is immobilization of the knee in an extension or cylinder cast for 4–6 weeks.
- **Club foot (talipes equinovarus)** is seen at birth. Both feet are turned inward, and there is plantar flexion of the ankle, inversion of the foot, adduction of the forefoot, and internal rotation of the tibia. Serial plaster casts started in the neonatal period provide sequential correction starting with the adducted forefoot, then the hindfoot varus, and last the equinus. About 50% of patients with club foot are fully corrected this way. The other 50% require surgery after age 6–8 months but before age <1–2 years.
- **Scoliosis** is seen primarily in adolescent girls whose thoracic spines are curved toward the right. The most sensitive screening finding is to look at the girl from behind while she bends forward, a hump will be noted over her right thorax. The deformity progresses until skeletal maturity is reached (at the onset of menses skeletal maturity is ~80%). In addition to the cosmetic deformity, severe cases develop decreased pulmonary function. Bracing is used to arrest progression; severe cases may require surgery. Early treatment is mandated.

Fractures

Remodeling occurs to an astonishing degree in children's fractures, thus degrees of angulation that would be unacceptable in the adult may be acceptable in children when these fractures are reduced and immobilized. Also, the healing process is much faster than in the adult. The only areas where children have special problems include supracondylar fractures of the humerus and fractures of any bone that involve the growth plate or epiphysis.

Supracondylar fractures of the humerus occur with hyperextension of the elbow in a child who falls on the hand with the arm extended. The injuries are particularly dangerous due to the proximity of the brachial artery and ulnar nerve. Although these fractures are treated with standard casting or traction and rarely need surgery), they require careful monitoring of vascular and nerve integrity and vigilance regarding development of compartment syndrome.

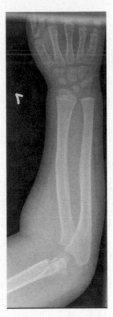

Figure I-2-1. Supracondular Fracture of the Humerus

Fractures that involve the **growth plate** or epiphysis can be treated by closed reduction if the epiphysis and growth plate are displaced laterally from the metaphysis but they are in one piece (i.e., the fracture does not cross the epiphysis or growth plate and does not involve the joint). If the growth plate is fractured into two pieces, open reduction and internal fixation will be required to ensure precise alignment and even growth to avoid chronic deformity of the extremity.

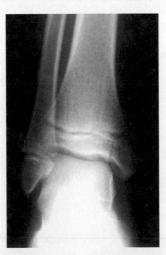

Figure I-2-2. Salter Harris Grade III Fracture

ADULT ORTHOPEDICS

X-rays for suspected fracture in adults should always include the following:

- Two views at 90° to one another
- Joints above and below the broken bone
- If suggested by the mechanism of injury, bones that are in "the line of force," which might also be broken (e.g. the lumbar spine must be evaluated for fracture following a fall from a significant height with foot fractures)

As a general rule, broken bones that are not badly displaced or angulated or that can be satisfactorily aligned by external manipulation can be immobilized in a cast ("closed reduction"). Broken bones that are severely displaced or angulated or that cannot be aligned easily require surgical intervention to reduce and fix the fracture ("open reduction and internal fixation").

Clavicular fracture is typically at the junction of middle and distal thirds. It is treated by placing the arm in a sling. Figure-of-8 bandage treatment is now less popular.

Anterior dislocation of the shoulder is by far the most common shoulder dislocation. Patients hold the arm close to their body but rotated outward as if they were going to shake hands. There may be numbness in a small area over the deltoid, from stretching of the axillary nerve. AP and lateral x-rays are diagnostic. Some patients develop recurrent dislocations with minimal trauma.

Posterior shoulder dislocation is rare and occurs after massive uncoordinated muscle contractions, such as epileptic seizure or electrical burn. The arm is held in the usual protective position (close to the body, internally rotated). Regular x-rays can easily miss it; axillary views or scapular lateral views are needed.

Colles' fracture results from a fall on an outstretched hand, often in old osteoporotic women. The deformed and painful wrist looks like a "dinner fork." The main lesion is an older, dorsally displaced, dorsally angulated fracture of the distal radius. Treatment is with close reduction and long arm cast.

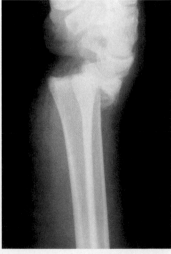

Figure I-2-3. X-ray demonstrating Colles Fracture with "Dinner-fork" Deformity

Monteggia fracture results from a direct blow to the ulna (i.e., on a raised protective arm hit by a nightstick). There is diaphyseal fracture of the proximal ulna, with anterior dislocation of the radial head. **Galeazzi fracture** is the mirror image: the distal third of the radius gets the direct blow and has the fracture, and there is dorsal dislocation of the distal radioulnar joint. In both of these, the broken bone often requires open reduction and internal fixation, whereas the dislocated one is typically handled with closed reduction.

Fracture of the scaphoid (carpal navicular) affects a young adult who falls on an out-stretched hand. Chief complaint is typically wrist pain, with physical exam revealing local-ized tenderness to palpation over the anatomic snuff box. In undisplaced fractures, x-rays are usually negative, but thumb spica cast is indicated just with the history and physical findings. X-rays will show the fracture 3 weeks later. If original x-rays show displaced and angulated fracture, open reduction and internal fixation are needed. Scaphoid fractures are notorious for a very high rate of nonunion secondary to avascular necrosis.

Metacarpal neck fracture (typically the fourth or fifth, or both) happens when a closed fist hits a hard surface (like a wall). The hand is swollen and tender, and x-rays are diagnostic. Treatment depends on the degree of angulation, displacement, or rotary malalignment: close reduction and ulnar gutter splint for the mild fractures, with Kirschner wire or plate fixation for bad ones.

Hip fracture typically occurs in the elderly following a fall. The hip hurts, and the patient's position in the stretcher is classic: the affected leg is shortened and externally rotated. Specific treatment depends on specific location (as shown by x-rays).

Femoral neck fracture, particularly if displaced, compromises the very tenuous blood supply of the femoral head. Faster healing and earlier mobilization can be achieved by replacing the femoral head with a prosthesis.

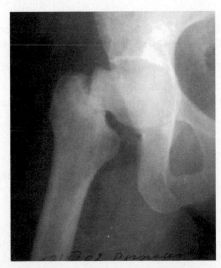

Reproduced with permission from the HWB Foundation,
www.hwbf.org/, courtesy of Dr. Alexander Chelnokov.

Figure I-2-4. Femoral Neck Fracture on X-ray of the Hip

Intertrochanteric fracture is less likely to lead to avascular necrosis, and is usually treated with open reduction and pinning. The unavoidable immobilization that ensues poses a very high risk for deep venous thrombosis and pulmonary emboli, thus post-op anticoagulation is recommended.

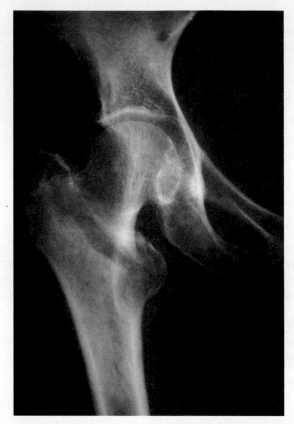

Figure I-2-5. Intertrochanteric Fracture of the Hip Noted on X-ray

Femoral shaft fracture is often treated with intramedullary rod fixation.

- If bilateral and comminuted, it may produce enough internal blood loss to lead to shock (external fixation may help while the patient is stabilized).

- If open, it is an orthopedic emergency, requiring OR irrigation and closure within 6 hours.

- If multiple, fat embolism syndrome may develop, in which severe respiratory distress occurs secondary to marrow fat entering the blood stream and embolizing to the pulmonary vasculature.

- Treatment is supportive care.

Knee injury typically produces swelling of the knee; knee pain without swelling is unlikely to be a serious knee injury. Collateral ligament injury is usually sustained when the force of impact is at the side of the knee, a common sports injury. Medial blows disrupt the lateral ligament and vice versa.

- The knee will be swollen and there is localized pain by direct palpation on the affected side.

- With the knee flexed 30°, passive abduction or adduction will produce pain on the torn ligaments and allow further displacement than the normal leg.

- Abduction demonstrates the medial injuries (valgus stress test), whereas adduction diagnoses the lateral injuries (varus stress test). Isolated injuries are treated with a hinged cast.
- When several ligaments are torn, surgical repair is preferred.

Anterior cruciate ligament injury is more common than posterior injury.

- There is severe knee swelling and pain.
- With the knee flexed 90°, the leg can be pulled anteriorly, like a drawer being opened (anterior drawer test).
- A similar finding can be elicited with the knee flexed at 20° by grasping the thigh with one hand, and pulling the leg with the other (Lachman test).

Posterior cruciate ligament injury produces the opposite findings. MRI is diagnostic. Sedentary patients may be treated with immobilization and rehabilitation, whereas athletes require arthroscopic reconstruction.

Meniscal tear is difficult to diagnose clinically and on x-rays, but is beautifully demonstrated on MRI.

- Protracted pain and swelling after a knee injury
- Possible "catching and locking," which limits knee motion, and a "click" when the knee is forcefully extended
- Repair is done, trying to save as much meniscus as possible
- Complete meniscectomy leads to the late development of degenerative arthritis

Injuries to the medial meniscus, medial collateral, and anterior cruciate often occur simultaneously.

Tibial stress fracture is seen in young men subjected to forced marches. There is tenderness to palpation over a very specific point on the bone, but x-rays are initially normal. Treat with a cast, and repeat the x-rays in 2 weeks. Non–weight bearing with crutches is another option.

Leg fracture involving the tibia and fibula is often seen when a pedestrian is hit by a car. Physical exam shows angulation; x-rays are diagnostic. Casting takes care of the ones that are easily reduced; intramedullary nailing is needed for the ones that cannot be aligned. The lower leg (along with the forearm) is one of the most common locations for development of the compartment syndrome. Increasing pain after a long leg cast has been applied always requires immediate removal of the cast and appropriate assessment.

Rupture of the Achilles tendon is seen in out-of-shape middle-aged men who subject themselves to severe strain (tennis, for instance). As they plant the foot and change direction, a loud popping noise is heard (like a rifle shot), and they fall clutching the ankle. Limited plantarflexion is still possible; but pain, swelling, and limping bring them to seek medical attention. Palpation of the tendon reveals a gap. Casting in equinus position allows healing in several months; surgery achieves a quicker cure.

Fracture of the ankle occurs when falling on an inverted or everted foot. In either case, both malleoli break. AP, lateral, and mortise x-rays are diagnostic. Open reduction and internal fixation are needed if the fragments are displaced.

Orthopedic Emergencies

Compartment syndrome occurs most frequently in the forearm or lower leg.

- Precipitating events include prolonged ischemia followed by reperfusion, crushing injuries, or other types of trauma.
- In the lower leg, by far the most common cause is a fracture with closed reduction.
- The patient has pain and limited use of the extremity; the compartment feels very tight and tender to palpation.
- The most reliable physical finding is excruciating pain with passive extension.
- Pulses may be normal.
- Emergency fasciotomy is required for treatment.

Pain under a cast is always handled by removing the cast and examining the limb.

Open fracture, in which a broken bone protrudes from the wound, requires irrigation in the OR and suitable reduction within 6 hours from the time of the injury. It is also called compound fracture.

Posterior dislocation of the hip occurs when the femur is driven backward, such as in a head-on car collision where the knees hit the dashboard. The patient has hip pain and lies in the stretcher with the leg shortened, adducted, and internally rotated (in a broken hip the leg is also shortened, but it is externally rotated). Because of the tenuous blood supply of the femoral head, emergency reduction is needed to avoid avascular necrosis.

Gas gangrene occurs with deep, penetrating, dirty wounds. In about 3 days the patient is extremely sick, looking toxic and moribund. The affected site is tender, swollen, discolored, and has gas crepitation. Treatment includes IV penicillin, extensive emergency surgical debridement, and possibly hyperbaric oxygen.

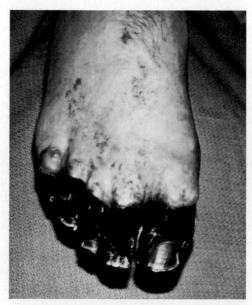

phil.cdc.gov

Figure I-2-6. Gangrene of the Toes

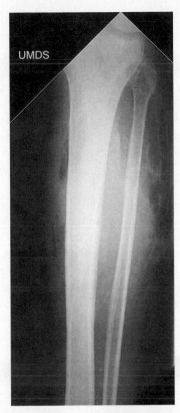

Reproduced with permission from SRS-X,
the SRS Educational Resource, the Scottish Radiological Society,
www.radiology.co.uk

Figure I-2-7. Gas Gangrene due to *Clostridium Perfringens* Infection

Associated neurovascular injuries

The **radial nerve** can be injured in oblique fractures of the middle to distal thirds of the humerus. If a patient comes in unable to dorsiflex (extend) the wrist, and regains function when the fracture is reduced and the arm is placed on a hanging cast or coaptation sling, no surgical exploration is needed. However, if nerve paralysis develops or remains after reduction, the nerve is entrapped and surgery has to be done.

Popliteal artery injury can occur in posterior dislocations of the knee. Following reduction of the dislocation, the popliteal artery must be evaluated with U/S, because even if distal pulses which had been absent return following reduction of the dislocation, there may be an intimal flap or local dissection that may need further evaluation with CT angiogram or surgical exploration. If pulses remain absent or an obvious injury is identified on U/S, surgical exploration is indicated. Delayed restoration of flow may require a prophylactic fasciotomy.

Injury patterns—the second hidden fracture

The direction of force that produces an obvious injury may produce another one that is less obvious and needs to be sought.

- **Falls from a height** landing on the feet may have obvious foot or leg fractures, but fractures of the lumbar or thoracic spine may be less obvious and must be assessed.

- **Head-on automobile collisions** may produce obvious injuries in the face, head, and torso, but if the knees hit the dashboard, the femoral heads may be driven backward into the pelvis or out of the acetabulum and thus cause a fracture or dislocation.

The presence of **facial fractures or closed head injuries** mandates evaluation of the cervical spine initially with CT scan and further with MRI if pain or neurological symptoms persist.

Common Hand Problems

Carpal tunnel syndrome occurs following performance of repetitive hand work such as typing and presents with numbness and tingling in both hands in the distribution of the median nerve (radial 3½ fingers). The symptoms can be reproduced by hanging the hand limply for a few minutes, or by tapping, percussing or pressing the median nerve over the carpal tunnel (Tinel's sign). The diagnosis is clinical, but the American Academy of Orthopaedic Surgery recommends that wrist x-rays (including carpal tunnel view) be done to rule out other pathology. Initial treatment is splinting and anti-inflammatory agents. If these conservative measures fail, surgery is indicated following electromyography and nerve conduction velocity.

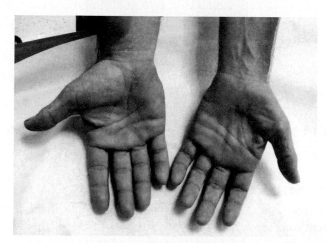

Figure I-2-8. Thenar Atrophy, a Feature of Carpal Tunnel Syndrome

Trigger finger is more common in women and presents with acute finger flexion and the inability to extend it unless pulled with the other hand, which results in a painful "snap." Steroid injection is the first line of therapy; surgery is the treatment of last resort.

De Quervain tenosynovitis is seen in young mothers who, as they carry their baby, force their hand into wrist flexion and thumb extension to hold the baby's head. They complain of pain along the radial side of the wrist and the first dorsal compartment. On physical exam the pain can be reproduced by asking her to hold the thumb inside her closed fist, then forcing the wrist into ulnar deviation. Splint and anti-inflammatory agents can help, but steroid injection is most effective. Surgery is rarely needed.

Dupuytren contracture occurs in older men of Norwegian ancestry and in alcoholics. There is contracture of the palm of the hand, and palmar fascial nodules can be felt. Surgery may be needed when the hand can no longer be placed flat on a table.

A **felon** is an abscess in the pulp of a fingertip, caused by a neglected penetrating injury. Patients complain of throbbing pain, and have all the classic findings of an abscess, including fever. Because the pulp is a closed space with multiple fascial trabecula, pressure can build up and lead to tissue necrosis; thus surgical drainage is urgently indicated.

Gamekeeper thumb is an injury of the ulnar collateral ligament sustained by forced hyper-extension of the thumb (historically suffered by gamekeepers when they killed rabbits by dislocating their necks with a violent blow with the extended thumb—nowadays seen as a skiing injury when the thumb gets stuck in the snow or the ski strap during a fall). On physical exam there is collateral laxity at the thumb-metacarpophalangeal joint, and if untreated it can be dysfunctional and painful, and lead to arthritis. Casting is usually effective.

Jersey finger is an injury to the flexor tendon sustained when the flexed finger is forcefully extended (as in someone unsuccessfully grabbing a running person by the jersey). When making a fist, the distal phalanx of the injured finger does not flex with the others.

Mallet finger is the opposite: the extended finger is forcefully flexed (a common volleyball injury), and the extensor tendon is ruptured. The tip of the affected finger remains flexed when the hand is extended, resembling a mallet. For both of these injuries, splinting is usually the first line of treatment.

Traumatically amputated digits are surgically reattached whenever possible. The amputated digit should be cleaned with sterile saline, wrapped in a saline-moistened gauze, placed in a sealed plastic bag, and the bag placed on a bed of ice. The digit should not be placed in antiseptic solutions or alcohol, should not be put on dry ice, and should not be allowed to freeze. With the use of electric nerve stimulation to preserve muscular function, entire amputated extremities can be reattached.

Back Pain

Lumbar disk herniation occurs most commonly at L4–L5 or L5–S1. Peak age incidence is the fourth decade of life.

- Patients often describe several months of vague aching pain (the "discogenic pain" produced by pressure on the anterior spinal ligament) before they have the sudden onset of the "neurogenic pain" precipitated by a forced movement.
- The latter is extremely severe, "like an electrical shock that shoots down the leg" (exiting on the side of the big toe in L4–L5, or the side of the little toe in L5–S1), and it is exacerbated by coughing, sneezing, or defecating (if the pain is not exacerbated by those activities, the problem is not a herniated disk). Patients cannot ambulate, and they hold the affected leg flexed.
- Straight leg-raising test reproduces excruciating pain and MRI confirms the diagnosis.
- Treatment for most patients is bed rest, physical therapy, and pain control, enhanced by a regional nerve block; surgical intervention is needed if neurologic deficits are progressing; emergency intervention is needed in the presence of the cauda equine syndrome (distended bladder, flaccid rectal sphincter, or perineal saddle anesthesia).

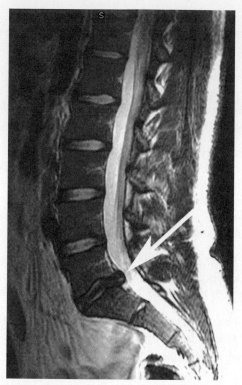

Figure I-2-9. Spine MRI Showing Lumbar
Disc Herniation of L4-L5 Interspace

Ankylosing spondylitis is seen in men in the third and fourth decades of life who complain of chronic back pain and morning stiffness. The pain is worse at rest, and improves with activity. Symptoms are progressive, and x-rays reveal a "bamboo spine." Anti-inflammatory agents and physical therapy are effective. Many of these patients have the HLA B-27 antigen, which is also associated with uveitis and inflammatory bowel disease.

Metastatic malignancy should be suspected in the elderly who have progressive back pain that is worse at night and unrelieved by rest or positional changes. Weight loss is often an additional finding. The most common pathology is lytic breast cancer metastases in women and blastic prostate metastases in men. Most lesions are identifiable on x-ray, but MRI is a more sensitive diagnostic tool.

Leg Ulcers

Diabetic ulcer is typically indolent and located at pressure points (heel and metatarsal head). It starts because of the neuropathy, and does not heal because of the microvascular disease. It can sometimes heal with good blood glucose control and wound care, but often becomes chronic and sometimes leads to amputation due to osteomyelitis.

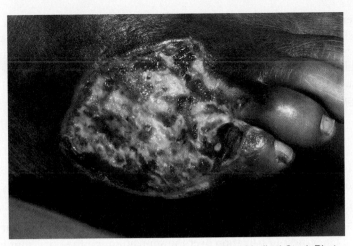

Figure I-2-10. Gross Appearance of a Large Diabetic Foot Ulcer

Ulcer from arterial insufficiency is usually as far away from the heart as it can be, i.e., at the tip of the toes. It looks dirty, with a pale base devoid of granulation tissue. The patient has other manifestations of arteriosclerotic occlusive disease (absent pulses, trophic changes, claudication, or rest pain). Workup begins with Doppler studies looking for a pressure gradient, though in the presence of microvascular disease this may not be present (and these lesions are less amenable to surgical therapy). Further evaluation with CT angiogram may be necessary, and ultimately, formal angiography leading to angioplasty, stenting, or surgical revascularization.

Venous stasis ulcer develops in chronically edematous, indurated, and hyperpigmented skin above the medial malleolus. The ulcer is painless, with a granulating bed. The patient has varicose veins, and suffers from frequent bouts of cellulitis. Duplex scan is useful in the workup. Treatment revolves around physical support to keep the veins empty: support stockings, Ace bandages, and Unna boots. Surgery may be required (vein stripping, grafting of the ulcer, injection sclerotherapy); endovascular ablation with laser or radiofrequency may also be used.

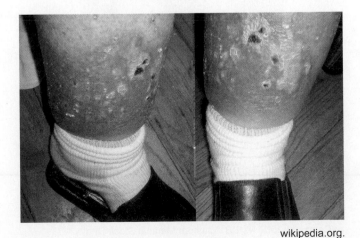

wikipedia.org.

Figure I-2-11. Venous Stasis Ulcers

Marjolin's ulcer is a squamous cell carcinoma of the skin that has developed in a chronic leg ulcer. The classic setting is one of many years of healing and breaking down, such as seen in untreated third-degree burns that underwent spontaneous healing, or in chronic draining sinuses secondary to osteomyelitis. A dirty-looking, deeper ulcer develops at the site, with heaped up tissue growth around the edges. Biopsy is diagnostic. Treatment is wide local excision and skin grafting if necessary.

Foot Pain

Plantar fasciitis is a very common but poorly understood problem affecting older, overweight patients who complain of disabling, sharp heel pain every time their foot strikes the ground.

- The pain is worse in the mornings.

- X-rays show a bony spur matching the location of the pain, and physical exam shows exquisite tenderness to palpation over the spur, although the bony spur is not likely the cause of the problem as many asymptomatic people have similar spurs.

- Spontaneous resolution occurs over several months, during which time symptomatic treatment is offered.

Morton's neuroma is an inflammation of the common digital nerve at the third interspace, between the third and fourth toes. The neuroma is palpable and exquisitely tender to palpation. The cause is typically the use of pointed, high heel shoes (or pointed cowboy boots) that force the toes to be bunched together. Management includes analgesics and more sensible shoes, but surgical excision can be performed if conservative management fails.

Gout typically produces swelling, redness, and exquisite pain of sudden onset at the first metatarsal-phalangeal joint in middle-aged obese men with high serum uric acid. Uric acid crystals are identified in fluid from the joint. Treatment for the acute attack is indomethacin and colchicine; treatment for chronic control is allopurinol and probenicid.

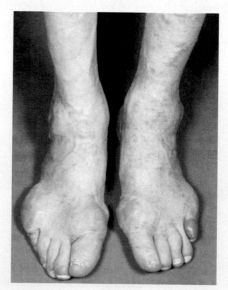

Copyright 2007 NMSB - Custom Medical Stock Photo.

Figure I-2-12. Gross Appearance of Acute Gout

TUMORS

Children and Young Adults

Primary malignant bone tumors are diseases of young people. They present with persistent low-grade pain for several months.

- **Osteogenic sarcoma** is the most common primary malignant bone tumor.
    - It is seen in ages 10–25, usually around the knee (lower femur or upper tibia).
    - A typical "sunburst" pattern is often described on x-rays.
- **Ewing sarcoma** is the second most common.
    - It affects younger children (ages 5–15) and it grows in the diaphyses of long bones.
    - A typical "onion skinning"–type pattern is often seen on x-rays.

Adults

Most malignant bone tumors in adults are metastatic, from the breast in women (lytic lesions) and from the prostate in men (blastic lesions). Localized pain is an early finding. X-rays can be diagnostic, CT scans give more information, and MRI is even more sensitive. Lytic lesions commonly present as pathologic fractures.

- **Multiple myeloma** is seen in old men and presents with fatigue, anemia, and localized pain at specific places on several bones. X-rays are diagnostic, showing multiple, punched-out lytic lesions.
    - They also have Bence-Jones protein in the urine and abnormal immunoglobulins in the blood, best demonstrated by serum protein electrophoresis (SPEP).
    - Treatment is chemotherapy; thalidomide can be used in the event that chemotherapy fails.
- **Soft tissue sarcoma** has relentless growth of soft tissue mass over several months. It is firm and typically fixed to surrounding structures.
    - It can metastasize hematogenously to the lungs but does not invade the lymphatic system.
    - MRI delineates the extent of the mass and invasion of local structures.
    - Incisional biopsy to obtain tissue is diagnostic.
    - Treatment includes wide local excision, radiation, and chemotherapy.

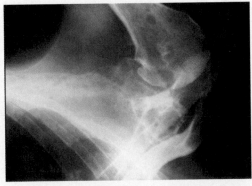

Figure I-2-13. Shoulder X-ray Showing
Punched-out Lesions of Multiple Myeloma

Learning Objectives

❑ List the appropriate steps in a preoperative assessment

❑ Recognize and describe the treatment approach to post-operative complications

PREOPERATIVE ASSESSMENT

Cardiac Risk

Ejection fraction <35% (normal 55%) poses prohibitive cardiac risk for elective non-cardiac operations. Incidence of peri-operative myocardial infarction (MI) could be as high as 75-85%, and mortality for such an event as high as 50–90%.

Goldman's index of cardiac risk assigns the following:

- 11 points to jugular venous distention (evidence of CHF)
- 10 points to recent MI (within 6 months)
- 7 points each to either premature ventricular contractions (≥5 per min) or a rhythm other than sinus rhythm
- 5 points to age >70
- 4 points to emergency nature of surgery
- 3 points each to either aortic valve stenosis, poor medical condition, or surgery within the chest or abdomen

The risk of life-threatening cardiac complications is only 1% with total score up to 5. The risk becomes 5% if the points total up to 12, increases to 11% with counts up to 25, and reaches 22% when the points >25.

Jugular venous distention, which indicates the presence of CHF, is the worst single finding predicting high cardiac risk. If at all possible, treatment with ACE inhibitors, beta-blockers, digitalis, and diuretics should precede surgery.

Recent MI is the next worse predictor of cardiac complications. Operative mortality within 3 months of the infarct is 40%, but drops to 6% after 6 months. Therefore delaying surgery longer than 6 months from MI is the best course of action. If surgery cannot be safely delayed, admission to the ICU before surgery is recommended to optimize cardiac performance.

Note

Do not memorize the specific percentages with respect to cardiac complications. Just get an idea of what contributes to cardiac risk.

Pulmonary Risk

Smoking is by far the most common cause of increased pulmonary risk, and the problem is compromised ventilation (high PCO_2, low forced expiratory volume in 1 second [FEV_1]), rather than compromised oxygenation. The smoking history, or the presence of chronic obstructive pulmonary disease (COPD), should lead to evaluation.

- Start with pulmonary function tests, and, if abnormal, obtain an arterial blood gas.
- Cessation of smoking for 8 weeks and intensive respiratory therapy (physical therapy, expectorants, incentive spirometry, humidified air) should precede surgery.

Hepatic Risk

Predictors of mortality are stratified by the Child-Pugh classification system. The contributing factors can be remembered as **A**scites, **B**ilirubin, **C**lotting (prothrombin time), **D**iet (serum albumin) and **E**ncephalopathy (presence/absence). Predict surgical mortality as follows:

- **~40% mortality** is predictable with bilirubin >2 mg/dL, albumin <3 g/dL, prothrombin time >16 sec, or encephalopathy.
- **~80–85% mortality** is predictable if 3 of the above are present (close to 100% if all 4 exist), or with either bilirubin alone >4 mg/dL, albumin <2 g/dL, or blood ammonia concentration >150 mg/dl.

Nutritional Risk

Severe nutritional depletion is identified by one or more of the following:

- Loss of 20% of body weight over 6 months
- Serum albumin <3 g/dL
- Anergy to skin antigens
- Serum transferrin level <200 mg/dl

Operative risk is multiplied significantly in those circumstances. Surprisingly, as few as 4–5 days of preoperative nutritional support (preferably via the gut) can make a big difference, and 7–10 days would be optimal if the surgery can be deferred for that long.

Metabolic Risk

Diabetic coma is an absolute contraindication to surgery. Rehydration, return of urinary output, and at least partial correction of the acidosis and hyperglycemia must be achieved before surgery.

POSTOPERATIVE COMPLICATIONS

Fever

Malignant hyperthermia develops shortly after the onset of the anesthetic (typically attributed to halothane or succinylcholine). Temperature >104°F and metabolic acidosis, hypercalcemia, and hyperkalemia also occur. A family history may exist. Treatment is IV dantrolene, 100% oxygen, correction of the acidosis, and cooling blankets. Monitor post-operatively for the development of myoglobinuria.

Bacteremia is seen within 30–45 minutes of invasive procedures (instrumentation of the urinary tract is a classic example), and presents as chills and a temperature spike as high as 104°F. Draw multiple sets of blood cultures and start empiric antibiotics.

Although rare, severe wound pain and very high fever within hours of surgery should alert you to the possibility of gas gangrene in the surgical wound. Immediately remove surgical dressings and examine the wound. Gas gangrene is not subtle, and should prompt immediate return to the OR for wound reopening and washout.

Postoperative fever 101–103° F is caused (sequentially in time) by atelectasis, pneumonia, UTI, deep venous thrombophlebitis, wound infection, or deep abscesses. ("wind, water, walking, wound")

Atelectasis is the most common source of fever on the first post-operative day. Assess the risk for the other causes listed above, listen to the lungs, do a chest x-ray, improve ventilation (deep breathing and coughing, postural drainage, incentive spirometry), and perform a bronchoscopy if necessary.

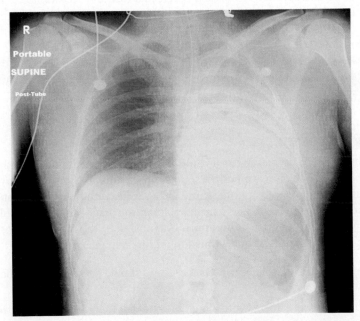

Copyright 2007 Bates, M.D. - Custom Medical Stock Photo.

Figure I-3-1. Total Left Sided Atelectasis

Pneumonia will happen in about 3 days if atelectasis is not resolved. Fever will persist, leukocytosis will be present, and chest x-ray will demonstrate an infiltrate(s). Obtain sputum cultures and treat with appropriate antibiotics.

UTI typically produces fever starting on post-operative day 3. Work up with a urinalysis and urinary cultures and treat with appropriate antibiotics.

Deep thrombophlebitis typically produces fever starting around post-operative day 5. Physical exam is not sensitive for this pathology, so obtain U/S with Doppler studies of the deep leg and pelvic veins. Treatment is systemic anticoagulation initially with heparin or unfractionated low molecular weight heparin and transitioned to a long term anticoagulant, typically Warfarin.

Wound infection typically begins to produce fever around post-operative day 7. Physical exam will reveal erythema, warmth, tenderness, and fluctuance.

- If only cellulitis is present, treat with antibiotics.
- If an abscess is present or suspected, the wound must be opened and drained.
- If it is unclear, use both U/S and CT scan to diagnose.

Deep abscesses (i.e. intra-peritoneal: subphrenic, pelvic, or subhepatic) start producing fever around post-operative days 10–15. CT scan of the appropriate body cavity is diagnostic. Percutaneous image-guided drainage is therapeutic.

Chest Pain

Perioperative myocardial infarction (MI) may occur during the operation (triggered most commonly by hypotension), in which case it is detected by the ECG monitor (ST depression, T-wave flattening). When it happens post-operatively, it is typically within the first 2–3 days, presenting as chest pain in one-third of patients and with the complications of the MI in the rest. The most reliable diagnostic test is serum troponin-I levels. Mortality is 50-90%and greatly exceeds that of MI not associated with surgery. Treatment is directed at the complications. Thrombolysis cannot be used in the peri-operative setting, but emergency angioplasty and coronary stenting can be life-saving.

Pulmonary Embolism

Pulmonary embolus (PE) typically occurs around post-operative day 7 in elderly and/or immobilized patients. The pain is pleuritic, sudden onset, and is accompanied by shortness of breath. The patient is anxious, diaphoretic, and tachycardic, with prominent distended veins in the neck and forehead (a low CVP virtually excludes the diagnosis). Arterial blood gases demonstrate hypoxemia and often hypocapnia. Diagnosis is with CT angiogram, which is a spiral CT with a large IV contrast bolus timed to pulmonary artery filling.

Treatment is systemic anticoagulation with heparin, and should be started immediately following diagnosis.

- In decompensating patients with a high index of suspicion, consider starting treatment even prior to confirming the diagnosis.
- If a PE recurs while anticoagulated or if anticoagulation is contraindicated, place an inferior vena cava (Greenfield) filter to prevent further embolization from lower extremity deep venous thromboses.

Prevention of thromboembolism will in turn prevent PE. Sequential compression devices should be used on anyone who does not have a lower extremity fracture or significant lower extremity arterial insufficiency. In moderate or high risk patients, prophylactic anticoagulation is indicated with lower dose heparin (typically 5000 units every 8-12 hours until mobile). Risk factors include age > 40, pelvic or leg fractures, venous injury, femoral venous catheter, and anticipated prolonged immobilization.

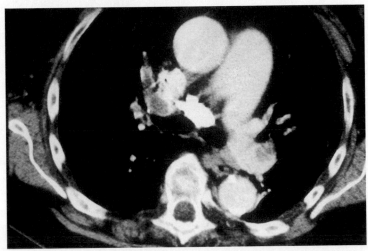

Copyright 2007 Bates, M.D. - Custom Medical Stock Photo.

Figure I-3-2. Spiral CT of Chest Demonstrating Pulmonary Embolus

Other Pulmonary Complications

Aspiration is a distinct hazard in awake intubations in combative patients with a full stomach. It can be lethal right away or lead to a chemical injury of the tracheobronchial tree and subsequent pulmonary failure and/or pneumonia. Prevention includes strict restriction of oral intake prior to surgery and antacids before induction. Therapy starts with bronchoscopic lavage and removal of acid and particulate matter followed by bronchodilators and respiratory support. Steroids usually don't help and so are not necessarily indicated. Antibiotics are only indicated if a patient demonstrates evidence of the resultant pneumonia, i.e. leukocytosis, sputum production and culture, and focal consolidation on chest x-ray.

Intraoperative tension pneumothorax can develop in patients with traumatized lungs once they are subjected to positive-pressure breathing. They become progressively more difficult to ventilate with rising airway pressure, BP steadily declines, and CVP steadily rises. If the abdomen is open, quick decompression can be achieved through the diaphragm but this is not recommended. A better approach is to place a needle through the anterior chest wall into the pleural space. Formal chest tube has to be placed following acute decompression.

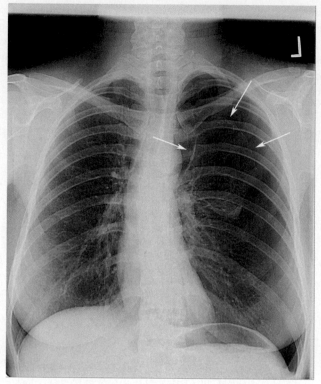

Figure I-3-3. Complete Left-sided Pneumothorax

Disorientation/Coma

Hypoxia is the first suspect when a post-operative patient becomes confused and disoriented. Sepsis is another prime cause. Check arterial blood gases and provide respiratory support if airway protection is threatened.

Adult respiratory distress syndrome (ARDS) is seen in patients with a complicated post-op course, often complicated by sepsis as the precipitating event. There are bilateral pulmonary infiltrates and hypoxia, with no evidence of CHF. The centerpiece of therapy is positive end-expiratory pressure (PEEP) with low volume ventilation as excessive ventilatory volumes have been demonstrated to result in barotrauma. A source of sepsis must be sought and corrected.

Delirium tremens (DTs) is very common in the alcoholic whose drinking is suddenly interrupted by surgery. During post-operative day 2 or 3, the patient gets confused, has hallucinations, and becomes combative. IV benzodiazepines are the standard therapy, but oral alcohol is available at most hospitals for this indication (less commonly used).

Acute hyponatremia can produce confusion, convulsions, and eventually coma and even death ("water intoxication"). This can be inadvertently induced by the liberal administration of sodium-free IV fluids (like D5W) in a postoperative patient with high levels of antidiuretic hormone (ADH; triggered by the response to trauma). Therapy, which includes hypertonic saline and osmotic diuretics, is controversial. Unfortunately mortality is high, especially in young women; the best management is prevention by including sodium in IV fluids.

Hypernatremia can also be a source of confusion, lethargy, and potentially coma, and rapidly induced by large, unreplaced water loss. Surgical damage to the posterior pituitary with unrecognized diabetes insipidus is a good example. Unrecognized osmotic diuresis can also do it. Rapid replacement of the fluid deficit is needed, but to "cushion" the impact on tonicity many prefer to use D51/2 or D51/3 normal saline (NS), rather than D5W.

Ammonium intoxication is a common source of coma in the cirrhotic patient with bleeding esophageal varices who undergoes a portocaval shunt.

Urinary Complications

Postoperative urinary retention is extremely common, particularly after surgery in the lower abdomen, pelvis, perineum, or groin. The patient feels the need to void, but cannot do it. Bladder catheterization should be performed 6-8 hours post-operatively if no spontaneous voiding has occurred. Indwelling (Foley) catheter placement is indicated at the second (some say third) consecutive catheterization.

Zero urinary output typically is caused by a mechanical problem, rather than a biologic one. Look for a plugged or kinked catheter, and flush the tubing to dislodge any clot that may have formed.

Low urinary output (<0.5 ml/kg/hr) in the presence of normal perfusing pressure (i.e., not because of shock) represents either fluid deficit or acute kidney injury.

- A low-tech diagnostic test is a fluid challenge: a bolus of 500 ml of IV fluid infused over 10 or 20 minutes. Dehydrated patients will respond with a temporary increase in urinary output, whereas those in renal failure will not do so.
- A more scientific test is to measure urinary sodium: it will be <10 or 20 mEq/L in the dehydrated patient with normally functional kidneys, while it will exceed 40 mEq/L in cases of renal failure.
- An even more scientific test is to calculate the fractional excretion of sodium, or FeNa. In order to calculate the FeNa, plasma and urinary sodium and creatinine must be measured. In acute kidney injury, the ratio >2; in hypovolemia it is <1.

Abdominal Distention

Paralytic ileus is to be expected in the first few days after abdominal surgery. Bowel sounds are absent or hypoactive and there is no passage of gas. There may be mild distension, but there is no pain. Paralytic ileus is prolonged by hypokalemia.

Early mechanical bowel obstruction because of adhesions can happen during the postoperative period. What was probably assumed to be paralytic ileus not resolving after 5-7 days is most likely an early mechanical bowel obstruction. X-rays will show dilated loops of small bowel and air-fluid levels. Diagnosis is confirmed with an abdominal CT scan that demonstrates a transition point between proximal dilated bowel and distal collapsed bowel at the site of the obstruction. Surgical intervention is needed to correct the problem.

Ogilvie syndrome or pseudo-obstruction is a poorly understood (but very common) condition that could be described as a "paralytic ileus of the colon."

- It does not follow abdominal surgery but is classically seen in elderly sedentary patients (Alzheimer, nursing home) who have become further immobilized owing to surgery elsewhere (broken hip, prostatic surgery).

- Patients develop abdominal distention without tenderness, and x-rays show a massively dilated colon.
- After fluid and electrolyte correction, it is imperative that mechanical obstruction be ruled out radiologically or by endoscopy, before giving IV neostigmine to restore colonic motility. A long rectal tube is also commonly used.
- This is a functional obstruction, not an anatomic one.

Wound

Wound infections are typically seen around post-operative day 7.

Wound dehiscence is typically seen around post-operative day 5 after open laparotomy. The wound looks intact, but large amounts of pink, "salmon-colored" fluid are noted to be soaking the dressing; this is peritoneal fluid. Reoperation is needed to avoid peritonitis and evisceration.

Evisceration is a catastrophic complication of wound dehiscence, where the skin itself opens up and the abdominal contents rush out. It typically happens when the patient (who may not have been recognized as having a dehiscence) coughs, strains, or gets out of bed. The patient must be kept in bed, and the bowel covered with large sterile dressings soaked with warm saline. Emergency abdominal closure is required.

Fistula of the GI tract is recognized because bowel contents leak out through a wound or drain site. It may harm the patient in a number of ways.

- If it does not empty completely to the outside but leaks into a cavity which then leaks out, an abscess may develop and lead to sepsis; complete drainage is the required treatment.
- If it drains freely, sepsis is not encountered (patient is typically afebrile with no signs of peritoneal irritation) though there are 3 other potential problems:
  - Fluid and electrolyte loss
  - Nutritional depletion
  - Erosion and digestion of the abdominal wall
- These problems are related to location and volume of the fistula:
  - Nonexistent in the distal colon
  - Present but manageable in low-volume fistula (up to 200–300 ml/day)
  - Upper GI fistulas (stomach, duodenum, upper jejunum)
  - Daunting in high-volume (several liters per day) fistulas in upper GI tract
- Fluid and electrolyte replacement, nutritional support (preferably elemental diets delivered beyond the fistula), and compulsive protection of the abdominal wall (frequent dressing changes, suction tubes, "ostomy" bags) are done to keep the patient alive until nature heals the fistula. Nature will do so if none of the following are present to prevent wound healing (**mnemonic: FRIENDS**):
  - Foreign body
  - Radiation injury
  - Infection or inflammatory bowel disease
  - Epithelialization
  - Neoplasm
  - Distal obstruction
  - Use of steroids

Fluids and Electrolytes

Hypernatremia invariably means that the patient has lost water (or other hypotonic fluids) and has developed hypertonicity. Every 3 mEq/L that the serum sodium concentration is >140 represents roughly 1 L of water lost.

- If the problem happens slowly (i.e., over several days), the brain will adapt and the only clinical manifestations will be those of volume depletion.

- Treatment requires volume repletion, but done in such a way that volume is corrected rapidly (in a matter of hours) while tonicity is only gently "nudged" in the right direction (and goes back to normal in a matter of days). This is achieved by using D51/2 NS rather than D5W.

- If the hypernatremia develops rapidly (i.e., in osmotic diuresis, or diabetes insipidus), it will produce CNS symptoms (the brain has not had time to adapt), and correction can be safely done with more diluted fluid (D51/3 NS, or even D5W).

Hyponatremia means that water has been retained and hypotonicity has developed, but there are 2 different scenarios (easily distinguishable by the clinical circumstances).

- In one scenario, a patient who starts with normal fluid volume adds to it by retaining water because of the presence of inappropriate amounts of ADH (e.g., post-op water intoxication, or inappropriate ADH secreted by tumors).

- In the other scenario, a patient who is losing large amounts of isotonic fluids (typically from the GI tract) is forced to retain water if he has not received appropriate replacement with isotonic fluids.

- Rapidly developing hyponatremia (water intoxication) produces CNS symptoms (the brain has not had time to adapt), and requires careful use of hypertonic saline (3% or 5%).

- In slowly developing hyponatremia from inappropriate ADH, the brain has time to adapt, and therapy should be water restriction.

- In the case of the hypovolemic, dehydrated patient losing GI fluids and forced to retain water, volume restoration with isotonic fluids (NS or Lactated Ringer's) will provide prompt correction of the hypovolemia and allow the body to slowly and safely unload the retained water and return the tonicity to normal.

Hypokalemia develops slowly (over days) when potassium is lost from the GI tract (all GI fluids have lots of K), or in the urine (because of loop diuretics, or too much aldosterone), and it is not replaced. Hypokalemia develops very rapidly (over hours) when potassium moves into the cells, most notably when diabetic ketoacidosis is corrected. Therapy is obviously potassium replacement. Remember that the safe "speed limit" of IV potassium administration is 10 mEq/hr.

Hyperkalemia will occur slowly if the kidney cannot excrete potassium (renal failure, aldosterone antagonists), and it will occur rapidly if potassium is being dumped from the cells into the blood (crushing injuries, dead tissue, acidosis). The ultimate therapy for hyperkalemia is hemodialysis, but while waiting for it we can help by "pushing potassium into the cells" (50% dextrose and insulin), sucking it out of the GI tract (NG suction, exchange resins such as Kayexelate if the patient's bowels are working), or neutralizing its effect on the cellular membrane (IV calcium). The latter provides the quickest protection.

Metabolic acidosis can occur from any of the following:

- Excessive production of fixed acids (diabetic ketoacidosis, lactic acidosis, low-flow states)
- Loss of buffers (loss of bicarbonate-rich fluids from the GI tract)
- Inability of the kidney to eliminate fixed acids (renal failure)

In all 3 cases, blood pH is low (<7.4), serum bicarbonate is low (<25), and there is a base deficit. When abnormal acids are piling up in the blood, there is also an "anion gap" (serum sodium exceeds by >10 or 15 the sum of chloride and bicarbonate), which does not exist when the problem is loss of buffers.

Treatment in all cases must be directed at the underlying cause, though in all cases administration of bicarbonate (or bicarbonate precursors, like lactate or acetate) would temporarily help correct the pH. Bicarbonate therapy, however, is ideal only when the initial problem is bicarbonate loss (it corrects the pH and it addresses the underlying problem). In other cases it risks producing a "rebound alkalosis" once the underlying problem is corrected. Thus correction of the underlying problem—rather than bicarbonate administration—is the preferred therapy. In long-standing acidosis, renal loss of K leads to a deficit that does not become obvious until the acidosis is corrected. One must be prepared to replace K as part of the therapy of acidosis.

Metabolic alkalosis occurs from loss of acid gastric juice, or from excessive administration of bicarbonate (or precursors). There is a high blood pH (>7.4), high serum bicarbonate (>25), and a base excess. In most cases, an abundant intake of KCl (5–10 mEq/h) will allow the kidney to correct the problem. Only rarely is ammonium chloride or 0.1 N HCl needed.

Respiratory acidosis and alkalosis result from impaired ventilation (acidosis) or abnormal hyperventilation (alkalosis). They are recognized by abnormal PCO_2 (low in alkalosis, high in acidosis) in conjunction with the abnormal pH of the blood. Therapy must be directed at improving ventilation (in acidosis) or reducing it (in alkalosis).

Learning Objectives

- ❏ Demonstrate understanding of surgical diseases of the gastrointestinal and endocrine systems
- ❏ Explain surgical treatment approaches for diseases of the breast
- ❏ Answer questions about surgical hypertension

DISEASES OF THE GASTROINTESTINAL SYSTEM

Upper Gastrointestinal System

Esophagus

Gastroesophageal reflux may produce vague symptoms, difficult to distinguish from other sources of epigastric distress. When the diagnosis is uncertain, pH monitoring is best to establish the presence of reflux and its correlation with the symptoms. In more typical cases, an overweight individual complains of burning retrosternal pain and "heartburn" that is brought about by bending over, wearing tight clothing, or lying flat in bed at night; it is relieved by the ingestion of antacids or over-the-counter H2 blockers. If there is a long-standing history, the concern is the damage that might have been done to the lower esophagus (peptic esophagitis) and the possible development of Barrett's esophagus. In that setting, endoscopy and biopsies are the indicated tests, as Barrett's is a precursor to malignancy.

Surgery for gastroesophageal reflux is:

- Appropriate in long-standing symptomatic disease that cannot be controlled by medical means (using laparoscopic Nissen fundoplication)
- Necessary when complications have developed (ulceration, stenosis) (using laparoscopic Nissen fundoplication)
- Imperative if there are severe dysplastic changes (resection is needed)

Motility problems have recognizable clinical patterns, such as crushing pain with swallowing in uncoordinated massive contraction, or the suggestive pattern of dysphagia seen in achalasia, where solids are swallowed with less difficulty than liquids. Manometry studies are used for the definitive diagnosis. Barium swallow is typically done first to evaluate for an obstructing lesion.

Achalasia is seen more commonly in women. There is dysphagia that is worse for liquids; the patient eventually learns that sitting up straight and waiting allows the weight of the column of liquid to overcome the sphincter. There is occasional regurgitation of undigested food.

X-rays show megaesophagus. Manometry is diagnostic. The most appealing current treatment is balloon dilatation done by endoscopy; however, recurrence is high and many patients ultimately require an esophagomyotomy (Heller).

Cancer of the esophagus shows the classic progression of dysphagia starting with meat, then other solids, then soft foods, eventually liquids, and finally (in several months) saliva. Significant weight loss is always seen. Squamous cell carcinoma is seen in men with a history of smoking and drinking. Adenocarcinoma is seen in people with long-standing gastroesophageal reflux. Diagnosis is established by endoscopy and biopsy. Endoscopic U/S and CT/PET scan are used to assess local and lymph node involvement and therefore operability, but most cases present late and therefore are inoperable.

Mallory-Weiss tear is a mucosal laceration typically at the junction of the esophagus and stomach. It occurs after prolonged, forceful vomiting and presents with bright red hematemesis. Endoscopy establishes diagnosis, and allows treatment with endoscopic clipping or coagulation.

Boerhaave's syndrome also results from prolonged, forceful vomiting but leads to esophageal perforation. There is continuous, severe, wrenching epigastric and low sternal pain of sudden onset, soon followed by fever, leukocytosis, and a very sick-looking patient. Contrast swallow (Gastrografin) is diagnostic, and emergency surgical repair should follow. Delay in diagnosis and treatment has grave consequences due to the morbidity of mediastinitis.

Instrumental perforation of the esophagus is by far the most common reason for esophageal perforation. Shortly after completion of endoscopy, symptoms as described above will develop. There may be emphysema in the lower neck (virtually diagnostic in this setting). Contrast studies and prompt repair are imperative.

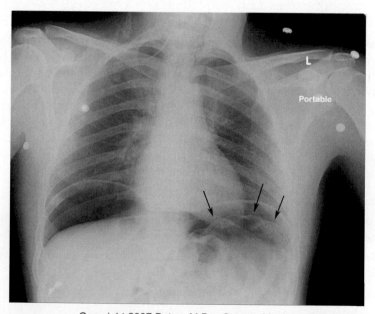

Copyright 2007 Bates, M.D. - Custom Medical Stock Photo.

Figure I-4-1. Upright Chest X-ray Demonstrating Free Air under the Diaphragm due to Colonic Perforation during Endoscopy

Stomach

Gastric adenocarcinoma is more common in the elderly. Symptoms include:

- Anorexia
- Weight loss
- Vague epigastric distress or early satiety
- Occasional hematemesis

Endoscopy and biopsies are diagnostic. CT scan helps assess operability. Surgery is the best therapy.

Gastric lymphoma is almost as common as gastric adenocarcinoma. Presentation and diagnosis are similar, but treatment is chemotherapy. Surgery is only indicated if perforation is feared as the tumor melts away. Low-grade lymphomatoid transformation (MALTOMA) can be reversed by eradication of *H. pylori*.

Mid and Lower Gastrointestinal System

Small bowel and appendix

Mechanical intestinal obstruction is typically caused by adhesions in those who have had a prior laparotomy. There is colicky abdominal pain and protracted vomiting, progressive abdominal distention (if it is a low obstruction), and no passage of gas or feces. Early on, high-pitched bowel sounds coincide with the colicky pain (after a few days there is silence). X-rays show distended loops of small bowel, with air-fluid levels. Treatment starts with NPO, NG suction, and IV fluids, hoping for spontaneous resolution, while watching for early signs of strangulation. Surgery is done if conservative management is unsuccessful, within 24 hours in cases of complete obstruction or within a few days in cases of partial obstruction.

Strangulated obstruction occurs due to compromised blood supply leading to bowel ischemia. It starts as described above, but eventually the patient develops fever, leukocytosis, constant pain, signs of peritoneal irritation, and ultimately full-blown peritonitis and sepsis. Emergency surgery is required.

Mechanical intestinal obstruction caused by an incarcerated hernia has the same clinical picture and potential for strangulation as described above, but the physical exam shows the irreducible hernia that used to be reducible. Because we can effectively eliminate the hernia (we cannot effectively eliminate adhesions), all of these undergo surgical repair, but the timing varies: emergently after proper rehydration in those who appear to be strangulated and electively in those who can be reduced manually and have a viable bowel.

Carcinoid syndrome is seen in patients with a small bowel carcinoid tumor with liver metastases. It includes diarrhea, flushing of the face, wheezing, and right-sided heart valvular damage (look for prominent jugular venous pulse). Diagnosis is made with 24-hour urinary collection for 5-hydroxyindolacetic acid.

(Hint: Whenever syndromes produce episodic attacks or spells, the offending agent will be at high concentrations in the blood only at the time of the attack. A blood sample taken afterward will be normal. Thus, a 24-hour urinary collection is more likely to provide the diagnosis.)

The **classic picture of acute appendicitis** begins with anorexia, followed by:

- Vague periumbilical pain that several hours later becomes sharp, severe, constant, and localized to the right lower quadrant of the abdomen

- Tenderness, guarding, and rebound found to the right and below the umbilicus (not elsewhere in the belly)

- Modest fever and leukocytosis in the 10,000–15,000 range, with neutrophilia and immature forms

Emergency appendectomy is the indicated treatment.

Doubtful presentations that could be acute appendicitis include those that do not have all the classic findings described above. CT scan has become the standard diagnostic modality for those cases.

Colon

Cancer of the right colon typically presents with anemia (hypochromic, iron deficiency) in the right age group (age 50–70). Stools will be 4+ for occult blood. Colonoscopy and biopsies are diagnostic; surgery (right hemicolectomy) is treatment of choice.

Cancer of the left colon typically presents with bloody bowel movements and obstruction. Blood coats the outside of the stool, there may be constipation, stools may have narrow caliber. Flexible proctosigmoidoscopic exam (45 or 60 cm) and biopsies are usually the first diagnostic study. Before surgery is done, full colonoscopy is needed to rule out a synchronous second primary lesion more proximally. CT scan helps assess operability and extent.

Colonic polyps may be premalignant. In descending order of probability for malignant degeneration are familial polyposis (and variants such as Gardner's), familial multiple inflammatory polyps, villous adenoma, and adenomatous polyp. Polyps that are not premalignant include juvenile, Peutz-Jeghers, isolated inflammatory, and hyperplastic.

Chronic ulcerative colitis (CUC) is managed medically. Surgical indications include disease present >20 years (high incidence of malignant degeneration), severe interference with nutritional status, multiple hospitalizations, need for high-dose steroids or immunosuppressants, or development of toxic megacolon (abdominal pain, fever, leukocytosis, epigastric tenderness, massively distended transverse colon on x-rays, with gas within the wall of the colon). Definitive surgical treatment of CUC requires removal of affected colon, including all of the rectal mucosa (which is always involved).

Pseudomembranous enterocolitis is caused by overgrowth of *Clostridium difficile* in patients who have been on antibiotics. Any antibiotic can do it. Clindamycin was the first one described, and, currently, Cephalosporins are the most common cause. There is profuse, watery diarrhea, crampy abdominal pain, fever, and leukocytosis. Diagnosis is best made by identifying the toxin in the stool. Stool cultures take too long, and the pseudomembranes are not always seen on endoscopy. The culpable antibiotic should be discontinued, and no antidiarrheals should be used. Metronidazole is the treatment of choice (oral or IV), with vancomycin (oral) an alternative. A virulent form of the disease, unresponsive to treatment, with WBC >50,000/μL and serum lactate above 5mg/dL, requires emergency colectomy.

Anorectal Disease

In **all anorectal disease, cancer should be ruled out** by proper physical exam (including proctosigmoidoscopic exam), even though the clinical presentation may suggest a specific benign process.

Hemorrhoids typically bleed when they are internal (can be treated with rubber band ligation), or hurt when they are external (may need surgery if conservative treatment fails). Internal hemorrhoids can become painful and produce itching if they are prolapsed.

Anal fissure happens to young women. There is exquisite pain with defecation and blood streaks covering the stools. The fear of pain is so intense that patients avoid bowel movements (and get constipated) and may even refuse proper physical examination of the area. Examination may need to be done under anesthesia (the fissure is usually posterior, in the midline). A tight sphincter is believed to cause and perpetuate the problem, thus therapy is directed at relaxing it: stool softeners, topical nitroglycerin, local injection of botulinum toxin, steroid suppositories, or lateral internal sphincterotomy. Calcium channel blockers such as diltiazem ointment 2% TID topically for 6 weeks have had an 80-90% success rate, as compared to only 50% success for botulinum toxin.

Crohn's disease often affects the anal area. It starts with a fissure, fistula, or small ulceration, but the diagnosis should be suspected when the area fails to heal and gets worse after surgical intervention (the anal area typically heals very well because it has excellent blood supply—failure to do so should suggest Crohn's disease). Surgery, in fact, should *not be done* in Crohn's disease of the anus. A fistula, if present, could be drained with setons while medical therapy is underway. Remicade helps healing.

Ischiorectal abscess (perirectal abscess) is very common. The patient is febrile, with exquisite perirectal pain that does not let him sit down or have bowel movements. Physical exam shows all the classic findings of an abscess (rubor, dolor, calor, and fluctuance) lateral to the anus, between the rectum and the ischial tuberosity. Incision and drainage are needed, and cancer should be ruled out by proper examination during the procedure. If patient is a poorly-controlled diabetic, necrotizing soft tissue infection may follow; significant monitoring is mandatory.

Fistula-in-ano develops in some patients who have had an ischiorectal abscess drained. Epithelial migration from the anal crypts (where the abscess originated) and from the perineal skin (where the drainage was done) form a permanent tract. Patient reports fecal soiling and occasional perineal discomfort. Physical exam shows an opening (or openings) lateral to the anus, a cordlike tract may be felt, and discharge may be expressed. Rule out a necrotic and draining tumor, and treat with fistulotomy.

Squamous cell carcinoma of the anus is more common in HIV, and in patients with receptive sexual practices. A fungating mass grows out of the anus, metastatic inguinal nodes are often felt. Diagnose with biopsy. Treatment starts with the Nigro chemoradiation protocol, followed by surgery if there is residual tumor. Currently the 5-week chemo-radiation protocol has a 90% success rate, so surgery is not commonly required.

Gastrointestinal Bleeding

General statistics of GI bleeding show that 3 of 4 cases originate in the upper GI tract (from the tip of the nose to the ligament of Treitz). One of 4 originates in the colon or rectum, and very few arise from the jejunum and ileum. GI bleeding arising from the colon comes from angiodysplasia, polyps, diverticulosis, or cancer, all of which are diseases of older people. Even hemorrhoids become more common with age. Therefore:

- When a young patient presents with GI bleed, the odds are overwhelming that it comes from the upper GI tract.

- When an older patient presents with GI bleed, it could be from anywhere (an "equal opportunity bleeder"), as the upper GI is the most common source overall (3/4), but age makes that old patient a good candidate for lower GI bleeding.

Vomiting blood always denotes a source in the upper GI tract. The same is true when blood is recovered by a NG tube in a patient who presents with bleeding per rectum. The best next diagnostic test in that setting is upper GI endoscopy. Be sure to look at the mouth and nose first.

Similarly, **melena** (black, tarry stool) always indicates digested blood, thus it must originate high enough to undergo digestion. Start the workup with upper GI endoscopy.

Red blood per rectum could come from anywhere in the GI tract (including upper GI, as it may have transited too fast to be digested). The first diagnostic maneuver if the patient is actively bleeding at the time is to pass an NG tube and aspirate gastric contents. If blood is retrieved, an upper source has been established (follow with upper endoscopy as above). If no blood is retrieved and the fluid is white (no bile), the territory from the tip of the nose to the pylorus has been excluded, but the duodenum is still a potential source and upper GI endoscopy is still necessary. If no blood is recovered and the fluid is green (bile tinged), the entire upper GI (tip of the nose to ligament of Treitz) has been excluded, and there is no need for an upper GI endoscopy.

Active bleeding per rectum, when upper GI has been excluded, is more difficult to work up. Bleeding hemorrhoids should always be excluded first by physical exam and anoscopy. Colonoscopy is not helpful during an active bleed as blood obscures the field. Once hemorrhoids have been excluded, management is based on the rate of bleeding.

- If the bleeding >2 mL/min (1 unit of blood every 4 hours), an angiogram is useful as it has a very good chance of finding the source and may allow for angiographic embolization.

- If the bleeding is slower, i.e. <0.5 mL/min, wait until the bleeding stops and then do a colonoscopy.

- For bleeding in between, do a tagged red-cell study

  - If the tagged blood collects somewhere indicating a site of bleeding, an angiogram may be productive.

    ° The curse of the tagged red-cell study is that it is a slow test, and by the time it is finished, the patient is often no longer bleeding and the subsequent angiogram is useless. In that case, at least there is some degree of localization of bleeding to indicate which side of the colon to resect if the patient rebleeds or emergently begins to exsanguinate.

  - If the tagged red cells do not show up on the scan, a subsequent colonoscopy is planned. Some practitioners always begin with the tagged red-cell study, regardless of the estimated rate of bleeding.

With increasing frequency in clinical practice, when bleeding is not found to be in the colon, capsule endoscopy is done to localize the spot in the small bowel. Of course this is done only when the patient is stable and upper and lower GI sources have been ruled out.

Patients with a recent history of blood per rectum, but not actively bleeding at the time of presentation, should start workup with upper GI endoscopy if they are young (overwhelming odds); but if they are old they need both an upper and a lower GI endoscopy (typically performed during the same session).

Blood per rectum in a child is most commonly a Meckel's diverticulum; start workup with a technetium scan looking for the ectopic gastric mucosa in the distal ileum.

Massive upper GI bleeding in the stressed, multiple trauma, or complicated post-op patient is probably from stress ulcers. Endoscopy will confirm. Angiographic embolization is the best therapeutic option. Better yet, they should be avoided by maintaining the gastric pH above 4 with prophylactic H2 blockers or proton pump inhibitors, which is now commonly done in the ICU setting.

Acute Abdomen

Acute abdominal pain can be caused by perforation, obstruction, or inflammatory/ischemic processes. Each of these groups has some common identifying characteristics.

- Acute abdominal pain caused by **perforation** has sudden onset and is constant, generalized, and very severe. The patient is reluctant to move, and very protective of his abdomen. Except in the very old or very sick, impressive generalized signs of peritoneal irritation are found: tenderness, muscle guarding, rebound, and lack of bowel sounds. Free air under the diaphragm on upright x-rays confirms the diagnosis. Perforated peptic ulcer is the most common example. Emergency surgery is indicated.

- Acute abdominal pain caused by **obstruction** of a narrow duct (ureter, cystic, or common bile) has sudden onset of colicky pain, with typical location and radiation according to source. The patient moves constantly, seeking a position of comfort. There are few physical findings, and they are limited to the area where the process is occurring.

- Acute abdominal pain caused by **inflammatory process** has gradual onset and slow buildup (at the very least a couple of hours, more commonly 6-12 hours). It is constant, starts as ill-defined and eventually localizes to the site of pathology, and often has typical radiation patterns. There are physical findings of peritoneal irritation in the affected area, and (except for pancreatitis) systemic signs such as fever and leukocytosis.

Ischemic processes affecting the bowel are the only ones that combine severe abdominal pain with blood in the lumen of the gut.

Spontaneous bacterial peritonitis (SBP) should be suspected in the child with nephrosis and ascites, or the adult with ascites who has a "mild" generalized acute abdomen with equivocal physical findings, and perhaps some fever and leukocytosis. Cultures of the ascitic fluid will yield a single organism (in garden-variety acute abdomens, a multiplicity of organisms grow). Treat with antibiotics, not with surgery.

Treatment for a generalized acute abdomen is exploratory laparotomy, with no need to have a specific diagnosis as to the exact nature of the process. With the exception of patients in whom SBP is suspected, other etiologies that mimic an acute abdomen must be ruled out before proceeding to exploration. These include myocardial ischemia (obtain an ECG), lower lobe pneumonia (perform a chest x-ray), PE (suspect in an immobilized patient), and abdominal processes that do not require surgical exploration, such as pancreatitis (check serum amylase and lipase) and urinary stones (perform a non-contrast CT scan of abdomen).

Acute pancreatitis should be suspected in the alcoholic who develops an "upper" acute abdomen. The classic picture has rapid onset for an inflammatory process (a few of hours), and the pain is constant, epigastric, radiating straight through to the back, with nausea, vomiting, and retching. Physical findings are relatively modest, found in the upper abdomen. Diagnose with serum amylase and lipase, CT if diagnosis is not clear. Treat with NPO, NG suction, IV fluids. (More details in pancreatic disease section.)

Biliary tract disease should be suspected in the obese multiparrous female patient ages 30-50 ("fat, female, forty, fertile") who presents with right upper quadrant abdominal pain.

Ureteral stones produce sudden onset colicky flank pain radiating to the inner thigh and scrotum or labia, sometimes with urinary symptoms like urgency and frequency; and with microhematuria discovered on urinalysis. Non-contrast CT scan is the best diagnostic test.

Acute diverticulitis is one of the very few inflammatory processes giving acute abdominal pain in the left lower quadrant (in women, the fallopian tube and ovary are other potential sources).

- Patients are typically middle-aged and present with fever, leukocytosis, physical findings of peritoneal irritation in the left lower quadrant, occasionally with a palpable tender mass.
- CT scan with oral and IV contrast is diagnostic.
- Treatment is NPO, IV fluids, and antibiotics.
- Most will cool down.
- Emergency surgery is needed for those who do not demonstrate evidence of free perforation of fistulization (most often to the bladder, presenting with pneumaturia).
- Radiologically guided percutaneous drainage of an abscess may be helpful and help prevent emergent surgical resection, but if successful, will usually require elective resection.
- Colonoscopy is indicated around 6 weeks after an episode of diverticulitis to rule out an underlying malignancy (endoscopy earlier in the presence of active inflammation increases the likelihood of perforation and decreases the diagnostic sensitivity).
- Elective resection of the involved colon is indicated for those who have had complications, multiple attacks, or continuing discomfort.

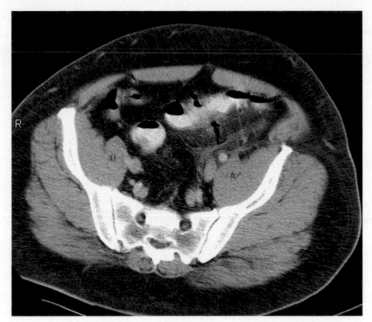

Copyright 2007 Bates, M.D. - Custom Medical Stock Photo.

Figure I-4-2. Abdominal CT scan of 56-year-old Man with
Acute Diverticulitis of Sigmoid Colon

Volvulus of the sigmoid is seen in older patients. It presents with signs of intestinal obstruction and severe abdominal distention. X-rays are diagnostic, as they show air-fluid levels in the small bowel, very distended colon, and a huge air-filled loop in the right upper quadrant that tapers down toward the left lower quadrant with the shape of a "parrot's beak."

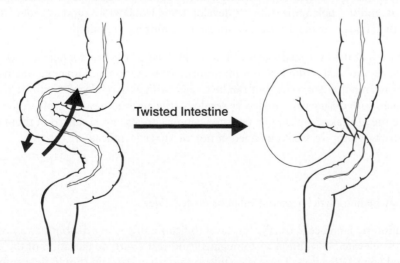

Twisted Intestine

Proctosigmoidoscopic exam resolves the acute problem and assesses for mucosal ischemia; leaving a rectal tube allows for complete decompression and prevents immediate recurrence. Recurrent cases need elective sigmoid resection.

Mesenteric ischemia is seen predominantly in the elderly, but the real key is the development of an acute abdomen in someone with atrial fibrillation or a recent MI (the source of the clot that breaks off and lodges in the superior mesenteric artery). Because the very old do not mount impressive acute abdomens, often the diagnosis is made late, when there is blood in the bowel lumen (the only condition that mixes acute pain with GI bleeding), and lactic acidosis and sepsis have developed. In very early cases, arteriogram and embolectomy might save the day, whereas once bowel ischemia is present, surgical resection is mandatory.

Hepatobiliary

Liver

Primary hepatoma (hepatocellular carcinoma) is seen in the United States in patients with cirrhosis. Patients develop vague right upper quadrant discomfort and weight loss. The specific blood marker is α-fetoprotein (AFP). CT scan will show location and extent. Resection is done if technically possible.

Metastatic cancer to the liver outnumbers primary cancer of the liver in the United States by 20:1. It is found by CT scan if follow-up for the treated primary tumor is under way, or suspected because of rising carcinoembryonic antigen (CEA) in those who had colonic cancer. If the primary is slow growing and the metastases are confined to one lobe, resection can be done. Other means of control include radiofrequency ablation (RFA).

Hepatic adenoma may arise as a complication of birth control pills, and is important because it has a tendency to rupture and bleed massively inside the abdomen. CT scan is diagnostic. If symptomatic, oral contraceptives should be stopped immediately; emergency surgery is required for patients presenting with signs of rupture and massive hemorrhage. Patients may not resume birth control pills.

Pyogenic liver abscess is seen most often as a complication of biliary tract disease, particularly acute ascending cholangitis. Patients develop fever, leukocytosis, and a tender liver. Sonogram or CT scan are diagnostic. Percutaneous drainage is required.

Amebic abscess of the liver favors men, all of whom have a "Mexico connection." (It is very common there, and seen in the U.S in immigrants.) Presentation and imaging diagnosis are similar to pyogenic liver abscesses, but can be treated with Metronidazole and rarely require drainage. Definitive diagnosis is maden by serology (the ameba does not grow in the pus), but because the test takes weeks to be reported, empiric treatment is started in those clinically suspected. If they improve, it is continued; if not, drainage is indicated.

Jaundice

Jaundice may be hemolytic, hepatocellular, or obstructive.

- **Hemolytic** jaundice is usually low level (bilirubin of 6-8 mg/dL, but not 35 or 40), and all the elevated bilirubin is unconjugated (indirect), with no elevation of the conjugated (direct) fraction. There is no bile in the urine. Workup should determine what is chewing up the red cells.
- **Hepatocellular** jaundice has elevations of both fractions of bilirubin, and very high levels of transaminases with only a modest elevation of the alkaline phosphatase. Hepatitis is the most common example, and workup should proceed in that direction (use serologies to determine specific type).

- **Obstructive** jaundice has elevations of both fractions of bilirubin, modest elevation of transaminases, and very high levels of alkaline phosphatase. The first step in the workup is an U/S looking for dilatation of the biliary ducts, as well as further clues as to the nature of the obstructive process. In obstruction caused by stones, the stone that is obstructing the common duct is seldom seen, but stones are seen in the gallbladder, which because of chronic irritation cannot dilate. In malignant obstruction, a large, thin-walled, distended gallbladder is often identified (Courvoisier-Terrier sign).

  - Obstructive jaundice caused by **stones** should be suspected in the obese, fecund woman in her forties, who has high alkaline phosphatase, dilated ducts on sonogram, and nondilated gallbladder full of stones. The next step in that case is an endoscopic retrograde cholangiopancreatography (ERCP) to confirm the diagnosis, perform a sphincterotomy, and remove the common duct stone. Cholecystectomy should usually follow during the same hospitalization.

  - Obstructive jaundice caused by a **tumor** could be caused by adenocarcinoma of the head of the pancreas, adenocarcinoma of the ampulla of Vater, or cholangiocarcinoma arising in the common duct itself.

    - Once a tumor has been suspected by the presence of dilated gallbladder in the sonogram, the next test should be CT scan. Pancreatic cancers that have produced obstructive jaundice are often big enough to be seen on CT. If the CT is negative, ERCP is the next step.

    - Ampullary cancers or cancers of the common duct by virtue of their strategic location produce obstruction when they are very small, and therefore may not be seen on CT. However, endoscopy will show ampullary cancers and the cholangiography will show intrinsic tumors arising from the duct (apple core) or small pancreatic cancers.

    - The recent advent of endoscopic U/S has given us another diagnostic pathway to locate and biopsy these tumors. Percutaneous biopsy is not indicated to avoid seeding the abdominal wall with tumor; if cancer is suspected and a tumor is identified on CT or ERCP, it should be resected if no contraindications are present (i.e. evidence of metastatic disease).

Ampullary cancer should be suspected when malignant obstructive jaundice coincides with anemia and positive blood in the stools.

- Can bleed into the lumen like any other mucosal malignancy, at the same time that it can obstruct biliary flow by virtue of its location.

- Given that combination, endoscopy should be the first test.

Pancreatic cancer is seldom cured, even when resectable by the Whipple operation (pancreatoduodenectomy).

Ampullary cancer and cancer of the lower end of the common duct have a much better prognosis (about 40% cure).

Gallbladder

Gallstones are responsible for the vast majority of biliary tract pathology. There is a spectrum of biliary disease caused by gallstones, as noted below. Although the obese woman in her forties is the "textbook" victim, incidence increases with age so that eventually they are common across all ethnic groups. Asymptomatic gallstones are left alone.

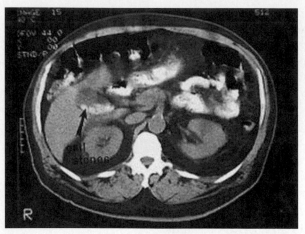

Figure I-4-3. Gallstones Noted on
CT Scan of Abdomen

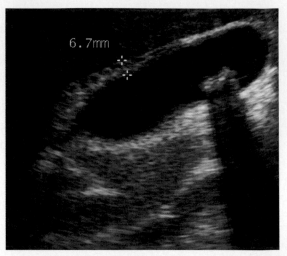

Figure I-4-4. Gallstones and a Thickened
Gallbladder Wall Noted on U/S

Biliary colic occurs when a stone temporarily occludes the cystic duct. This causes colicky pain in the right upper quadrant radiating to the right shoulder and back, often triggered by ingestion of fatty food, accompanied by nausea and vomiting, but without signs of peritoneal irritation or systemic signs of inflammatory process. The episode is self-limited (10, 20, maybe 30 minutes), or easily aborted by anticholinergics. U/S establishes diagnosis of gallstones and elective laparoscopic cholecystectomy is indicated.

Acute cholecystitis starts as a biliary colic, but the stone remains at the cystic duct until an inflammatory process develops in the obstructed gallbladder.

- Pain becomes constant, there is modest fever and leukocytosis, and there are physical findings of peritoneal irritation in the right upper quadrant.
- Liver function tests are minimally affected.
- U/S is diagnostic in most cases (gallstones, thick-walled gallbladder, and pericholecystic fluid).
- In equivocal cases, a radionuclide scan (HIDA) might be needed, and would show tracer uptake in the liver, common duct, and duodenum, but not in the occluded gallbladder.
- NPO, IV fluids, and antibiotics "cool down" most cases, allowing elective laparoscopic cholecystectomy to follow.
- Physicians typically endeavor to do it in the same hospital admission, as an urgent case, though it is not a "middle of the night" true emergency.
- If the patient doesn't respond (men and diabetics often do not), emergency cholecystectomy will be needed. Emergency percutaneous cholecystostomy may be the best temporizing option in the very sick with a prohibitive surgical risk.

Acute ascending cholangitis is a far more deadly disease, in which stones have reached the common duct producing partial obstruction and ascending infection.

- Patients are often older and much sicker.
- Temperature spikes to 104–105°F, with chills, and very high white blood cell count indicates sepsis.
- There is some hyperbilirubinemia but the key finding is extremely high levels of alkaline phosphatase.
- Charcot's triad is the presence of fever, jaundice, and right upper quadrant pain and is suggestive of ascending cholangitis; Reynolds pentad is those 3 symptoms plus altered mental status and evidence of sepsis (most commonly, hypotension), which further suggests the diagnosis.
- IV antibiotics and emergency decompression of the common duct is lifesaving; this is performed ideally by ERCP, alternatively percutaneous through the liver by percutaneous transhepatic cholangiogram (PTC), or rarely by surgery.
- Eventually, cholecystectomy has to be performed.

Obstructive jaundice without ascending cholangitis can occur when stones produce complete biliary obstruction, rather than partial obstruction. Presentation and management were detailed in the jaundice section.

Biliary pancreatitis is seen when stones become impacted distally in the ampulla, temporarily obstructing both pancreatic and biliary ducts. The stones often pass spontaneously, producing a mild and transitory episode of cholangitis along with the classic manifestations of pancreatitis (elevated amylase or lipase). U/S confirms gallstones in the gallbladder. Medical management (NPO, NG suction, IV fluids) usually leads to improvement, allowing elective cholecystectomy to be done later. If not, ERCP and sphincterotomy may be required to dislodge the impacted stone.

Pancreas

Acute pancreatitis is seen as a complication of gallstones (as described above), or in alcoholics. Acute pancreatitis may be edematous, hemorrhagic, or suppurative (pancreatic abscess). Late complications include pancreatic pseudocyst and chronic pancreatitis.

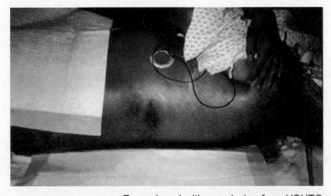

Reproduced with permission from VGHTC,
Gastroenterology Section.

Figure I-4-5. Grey-Turner Sign Can Be
seen in Acute Pancreatitis

Acute edematous pancreatitis occurs in the alcoholic or the patient with gallstones. Epigastric and midabdominal pain starts after a heavy meal or bout of alcoholic intake, is constant, radiates straight through to the back, and is accompanied by nausea, vomiting, and (after the stomach is empty) continued retching. There is tenderness and mild rebound in the upper abdomen. Serum amylase and lipase are elevated, and often serum hematocrit levels are high due to hypovolemia. Resolution usually follows a few days of pancreatic rest (NPO, NG suction, IV fluids).

Acute severe pancreatitis is a much more deadly disease. It starts as the edematous form does, but an early lab clue is lower hematocrit (the degree of amylase elevation does not correlate with the severity of the disease). Other findings have been catalogued (Ranson's criteria):

- At the time of presentation, elevated WBC count, elevated blood glucose, and low serum calcium
- By the next morning, hematocrit is even lower, continued low serum calcium (in spite of calcium administration), increased blood urea nitrogen, and eventual metabolic acidosis and low arterial PO_2

Prognosis at that time is terrible, and intensive supportive therapy is needed in the ICU. This includes significant IV fluid hydration, possibly mechanical ventilation, and enteral feeding (distal to the pancreas). A common final pathway for death is the development of multiple pancreatic abscesses; try to anticipate them and drain if possible. If drained fluid is positive for bacteria (often gram-negative), the antibiotic of choice is IV carbopenem (imipenem or meropenem).

Necrosectomy is the best way to deal with necrotic pancreas, but timing is crucial. Most practitioners will wait as long as possible before necrosectomy is offered, as it requires the dead tissue to delineate well and mature for dissection. Patients do far better by waiting at least 4 weeks before debridement of the dead pancreatic tissue. Many pancreatic abscesses are not amenable to percutaneous or open drainage and will require open drainage or debridement.

Pancreatic abscess (acute suppurative pancreatitis) may become evident in someone who was not getting CT scans, because persistent fever and leukocytosis develop ~10 days after the onset of pancreatitis and sepsis develops. Imaging studies done at that time will reveal the collection(s) of pus, and percutaneous drainage and imipenem or meropenem will be indicated.

Pancreatic pseudocyst can be a late sequela of acute pancreatitis, or of pancreatic (upper abdominal) trauma. In either case, ~5 weeks elapses between the original problem and the discovery of the pseudocyst. There is a collection of pancreatic juice outside the pancreatic ducts (most commonly in the lesser sac), and the pressure symptoms thereof (early satiety, vague symptoms, discomfort, a deep palpable mass). CT or U/S will be diagnostic. Treatment is dictated by the size and age of the pseudocyst.

- Cysts ≤6 cm or those that have been present <6 weeks are not likely to have complications and can be observed for spontaneous resolution.
- Larger (>6 cm) or older cysts (>6 weeks) are more likely to cause obstruction, bleed, or get infected, and they need to be treated.

Treatment involves drainage of the cyst. The cyst can be drained percutaneously to the outside, drained surgically into the GI tract, or drained endoscopically into the stomach.

Chronic pancreatitis is a devastating disease. People who have repeated episodes of pancreatitis (usually alcoholic) eventually develop calcified burned-out pancreas, steatorrhea, diabetes, and constant epigastric pain. The diabetes and steatorrhea can be controlled with insulin and pancreatic enzymes, but the pain is resistant to most modalities of therapy and can be incredibly debilitating. If ERCP shows specific points of obstruction and dilatation, operations that drain the pancreatic duct may help.

Hernias

All abdominal hernias should be electively repaired to avoid the risk of intestinal obstruction and strangulation. Exceptions include:

- Asymptomatic umbilical hernia in patients age <5 (they typically close spontaneously)
- Esophageal sliding hiatal hernias (not "true" hernias)

Hernias that become irreducible need emergency surgery to prevent strangulation. Those that have been irreducible for years need elective repair.

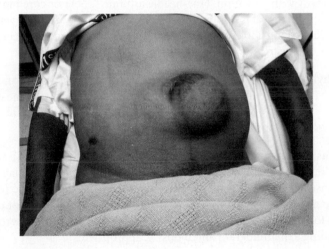

Figure I-4-6. Gross Appearance of Large Umbilical Hernia

DISEASES OF THE BREAST

In all breast disease, cancer must be ruled out even if the presentation initially suggests benign disease. The only sure way to rule out cancer is to get tissue for the pathologist. Age correlates best with the odds for cancer:

- Virtually unknown in the teens
- Rare in young women
- Quite possible by middle age
- Very likely in the elderly

Women with a family history are at greater risk from an earlier age.

Mammography is not a substitute for tissue diagnosis, but is an important adjunct to physical examination. A breast mass that might be missed by palpation may be seen on mammogram, and the opposite can also be true.

- As a regular screening exam, mammography should be started between ages 40-50 (earlier if there is family history).

- Mammography is not as helpful in women age <30 (breast is too dense) or during lactation (increased parenchymal density). In these cases, ultrasound is often used to work-up breast complaints. Mammography can be done if necessary during pregnancy.

- Stereotactic (i.e. mammogram-directed core needle biopsy) or U/S-guided core biopsies have become the most convenient, effective, and inexpensive way to biopsy breast masses, whether they are palpable or are discovered by screening mammogram.

- Annual MRI screening, in addition to mammography, may be considered in patients with significant risk factors for developing breast cancer (e.g., BRCA, mediastinal irradiation for Hodgkins age 10-30, significant family history risk).

Fibroadenoma is primarily seen in young women (late teens, 20s, or 30s) as a firm, rubbery mass that moves easily with palpation. Fine-needle aspirate (FNA) or core biopsy is sufficient to establish diagnosis. Removal is optional in uncomplicated cases. Giant juvenile fibroadenoma is seen in very young adolescents, where it has very rapid growth. Removal is needed to avoid deformity and distortion of the breast.

Cystosarcoma phyllodes tumors are most common in women in their 30s and 40s, but women of any age can have them. They can become very large, distorting the entire breast, yet not invading or becoming fixed. Most are benign, but a malignant variant is also possible. Core biopsy is needed (FNA is not sufficient), and removal is mandatory.

Mammary dysplasia (fibrocystic disease, cystic mastitis) is most common in women of childbearing age, but can affect women of any age. It often presents with bilateral tenderness related to the menstrual cycle and multiple lumps that seem to come and go (they are cysts) also following the menstrual cycle. Ultrasound can be used to evaluate breast complaints and is also diagnostic for simple cysts. Any dominant or persistent mass of concern should be worked-up, including a mammogram and biopsy if appropriate.

Intraductal papilloma is seen in women with bloody nipple discharge. Mammogram is needed to exclude other potential lesions, but it will not show the papilloma (they are tiny). Galactogram or U/S may be diagnostic and guide surgical resection. However, any patient with a bloody nipple discharge is cancer until proven otherwise.

Mastititis and **breast abscesses** are most commonly seen in lactating women; what appears to be a breast abscess at other times is cancer until proven otherwise. Mastitis is treated with oral antibiotics alone, whereas ultrasound-guided fine needle aspiration or incision and drainage are needed to drain a true abscess.

Breast cancer should be suspected in any woman with a palpable breast mass, and the index of suspicion increases with the patient's age. Other strong indicators of cancer include:

- Ill-defined fixed mass
- Retraction of overlying skin
- Recent retraction of the nipple
- Eczematoid lesions of the areola
- Reddish orange peel skin over the mass (inflammatory cancer)
- Palpable axillary nodes

A history of trauma does not rule out cancer.

Breast cancer during pregnancy is diagnosed exactly as if pregnancy did not exist, and is treated the same way with the following exceptions:

- No radiotherapy during the pregnancy
- No chemotherapy during the first trimester

Termination of the pregnancy is not necessary.

The radiologic appearance of breast cancer on mammogram includes an irregular, speculated mass, asymmetric density, architectural distortion or fine microcalcifications that were not there in a previous study.

Treatment of resectable breast cancer starts with lumpectomy (partial mastectomy) plus post-op radiation or total mastectomy; either way, axillary sentinel lymph node sampling is performed simultaneously. The sentinel node biopsy is performed only when nodes are not palpable on physical exam. Lumpectomy is an ideal option when the tumor is small, not multicentric, and not associated with extensive DCIS.

Infiltrating (or invasive) ductal carcinoma is the common standard form of breast cancer. Other variants (lobular, medullary, tubular, mucinous) tend to have slightly better prognosis, and are treated the same way as the standard infiltrating ductal. Lobular has higher incidence of bilaterality.

Inflammatory cancer is a clinical presentation of advanced breast cancer. It has a much worse prognosis and is treated with chemotherapy prior to surgery. The surgery for inflammatory breast cancer is almost always a modified radical mastectomy. Inflammatory breast cancer is also one of the few times where radiation is added following a total mastectomy. It mimics mastitis but is not an infectious process, and antibiotics do not play a role in treatment.

Ductal carcinoma in situ is a precursor to invasive breast cancer. Since it is confined to the ducts, it cannot metastasize (thus no axillary sampling is needed). Total mastectomy is recommended for multicentric lesions throughout the breast; many practitioners add a sentinel node biopsy in those patients, in the event that invasive cancer is found following the mastectomy, as a sentinel node cannot be done after the breast has been removed. Lumpectomy with or without radiation is used if the lesion(s) are confined to a limited portion of the breast.

Inoperable cancer of the breast is breast cancer that is not amenable to surgical resection. Inoperability is based primarily on local extent (not metastases). Treatment for inoperable breast cancer can include any combination of chemotherapy, hormone therapy (if hormone receptor positive), or radiation, and is often considered palliative. In some cases, chemotherapy may shrink the cancer making it feasible for surgery.

Adjuvant systemic therapy may follow surgery, particularly if the tumor is >1cm, high-grade, HER2 positive, or axillary nodes are positive. Anti-estrogen hormonal therapy is an option for adjuvant systemic therapy if the tumor is receptor-positive. Women with small, low-risk tumors may be offered hormonal therapy alone (i.e. without chemotherapy) if their tumors are estrogen-receptor positive.

- Premenopausal women receive tamoxifen
- Postmenopausal women receive an aromatase-inhibitor (e.g. anastrozole)

Persistent headache or back pain (with areas of localized tenderness) in women who recently had breast cancer suggests metastasis. MRI is diagnostic – other tests for spine metastasis may include bone scan, CT scan, and PET. Brain metastases can be radiated or resected. The vertebral body and pedicles are the favorite location in the spine.

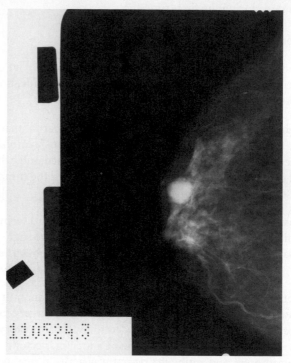

visualsonline.cancer.gov

Figure I-4-7. Large Calcification Located within a Case of Overt Breast Cancer Noted on Mammography

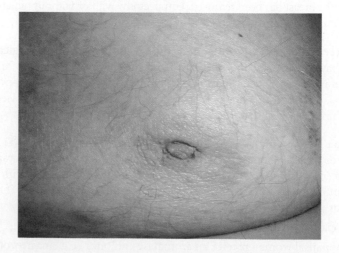

Figure I-4-8. Peau d'Orange is Seen in Some Cases of Breast Cancer

DISEASES OF THE ENDOCRINE SYSTEM

Thyroid nodules in euthyroid patients could be cancer, but incidence is low and indiscriminate thyroidectomy is not justified. FNA is the diagnostic method of choice.

- If read as benign, continue to follow the patient but do not intervene.
- If read as malignant or indeterminate, follow with a thyroid lobectomy.
- The need for further surgery is determined by the histologic diagnosis given from a frozen section.
- A total thyroidectomy should be performed in follicular cancers, so that if needed, radioactive iodine can be used in the future to treat blood-borne metastases.

Thyroid nodules in hyperthyroid patients are almost never cancer, but they may be the source of the hyperfunction ("hot adenomas"). Clinical signs of hyperthyroidism include:

- Weight loss in spite of ravenous appetite
- Palpitations
- Heat intolerance
- Moist skin
- Fidgety and hyperactive behavior
- Tachycardia
- Atrial fibrillation or flutter (occasional)

Laboratory confirmation can be done with thyrotropin (TSH; low) or thyroxine (T4; high). Nuclear scan will show if the nodule is the source. Most hyperthyroid patients are treated with radioactive iodine, but those with a "hot adenoma" have the option of surgical excision of the affected lobe.

Hyperparathyroidism is most commonly found by serendipitous discovery of high serum calcium in blood tests (rarely seen in the full florid "disease of stones, bones, and abdominal groans"). Repeat calcium determinations, look for low phosphorus, and rule out cancer with bone metastases. If findings persist, do parathyroid hormone (PTH) determination (and interpret in light of serum calcium levels).

- Asymptomatic patients become symptomatic at a rate of 20% per year; thus elective intervention is justified.
- Ninety percent have single adenoma.
- Removal is curative (sestamibi scan may help localize the culprit gland before surgery).

Cushing's syndrome presents with a round, ruddy, hairy face, buffalo hump, supraclavicular fat pads, obese trunk with abdominal stria, and thin weak extremities, classically in a patient with a normal previous appearance. Osteoporosis, diabetes, hypertension, and mental instability are also present. Workup starts with an overnight low-dose dexamethasone suppression test.

- Suppression at low dosage rules out the disease.
- If no suppression, measure 24-hour urine-free cortisol; if elevated, move to a high-dose suppression test.
  - Suppression at a higher dose identifies pituitary microadenoma.
  - No suppression at higher dose identifies adrenal adenoma (or paraneoplastic syndrome).
- Do appropriate imaging studies (MRI for pituitary, CT scan for adrenal) and remove the offending adenoma.

Zollinger-Ellison syndrome (gastrinoma) shows up as virulent peptic ulcer disease, resistant to all usual therapy (including eradication of *Helicobacter pylori*), and more extensive than it should be (several ulcers rather than one, ulcers extending beyond first portion of the duodenum). Some patients also have watery diarrhea. Measure gastrin and do a secretin test; if values are equivocal, locate the tumor with CT scan (with contrast) of the pancreas and nearby areas and resect it. Omeprazole helps those with metastatic disease.

Insulinoma produces CNS symptoms because of low blood sugar, always when the patient is fasting. Differential diagnosis is with reactive hypoglycemia (attacks occur after eating), and with self-administration of insulin. In the latter the patient has reason to be familiar with insulin (some connection with the medical profession, or with a diabetic patient), and in plasma assays has high insulin but low C-peptide. In insulinom, both are high. Do CT (with contrast) of the pancreas to locate the tumor and then resect it. Glucagonoma produces severe migratory necrolytic dermatitis, resistant to all forms of therapy, in a patient with mild diabetes, mild anemia, glossitis, and stomatitis. Glucagon assay is diagnostic, CT scan is used to locate the tumor, resection is curative. Somatostatin and streptozocin can help those with metastatic, inoperable disease.

SURGICAL HYPERTENSION

Primary hyperaldosteronism can be caused by an adenoma or by hyperplasia. In both cases the key finding is hypokalemia in a hypertensive (usually female) patient who is not on diuretics. Other findings include modest hypernatremia and metabolic alkalosis. Aldosterone levels are high, whereas renin levels are low. Appropriate response to postural changes (more aldosterone when upright than when lying down) suggests hyperplasia (which is treated medically), whereas lack of response (or inappropriate response) is diagnostic of adenoma. Adrenal CT scans localize it, and surgical removal provides cure.

Pheochromocytoma is seen in thin, hyperactive women who have attacks of pounding headache, perspiration, palpitations, and pallor (i.e., extremely high but paroxysmal BP). By the time patients are seen, the attack has subsided and pressure may be normal, leading to a frustrating lack of diagnosis. Patients who have sustained hypertension are easier to diagnose.

- Start the workup with a 24-hour urinary determination of vanillylmandelic acid (VMA), metanephrines (more specific), or free urinary catecholamines.
- Follow with a CT scan of the adrenal glands and retroperitoneum; if negative, a radionuclide study may be necessary to identify extra-adrenal sites.
- Tumors are usually large.
- Surgery requires careful pharmacologic preparation with alpha-blockers, followed by beta-blockers.

Coarctation of the aorta may be recognized at any age, but patients are typically young and have hypertension in the arms, with normal pressure (or low pressure, or no clinical pulses) in the lower extremities. Chest x-ray shows scalloping of the ribs (erosion from large collateral intercostals). CT angiogram (CTA) is diagnostic and surgical correction is curative.

Renovascular hypertension is seen in 2 distinct groups: **young women with fibromuscular dysplasia,** and **old men with arteriosclerotic occlusive disease**.

In both groups hypertension is resistant to the usual medications, and a telltale faint bruit over the flank or upper abdomen suggests the diagnosis. Workup is multifactorial, but Duplex scan of the renal vessels and CTA have prominent roles. Therapy is imperative in the young women—usually balloon dilatation and stenting—but it is much more controversial in the old men who may have short life expectancy from the other manifestations of the arteriosclerosis.

Pediatric Surgery 5

Learning Objectives

❑　Demonstrate understanding of common surgical problems in children within the first 24 hours of birth, within the first 2 months of life, and later in infancy

BIRTH—FIRST 24 HOURS

Most congenital anomalies require surgical correction, but in most of them other anomalies have to be looked for first. In some cases clusters are seen.

Esophageal atresia presents with excessive salivation noted shortly after birth or choking spells when first feeding is attempted. A small NG tube is passed, and it will be seen coiled in the upper chest when x-rays are done. If there is normal gas pattern in the bowel, the baby has the most common form of the 4 types, in which there is a blind pouch in the upper esophagus and a fistula between the lower esophagus and the tracheobronchial tree.

Before therapy is undertaken, rule out associated anomalies (the vertebral, anal, cardiac, tracheal, esophageal, renal, and radial [VACTER] constellation):

- Look at the anus for imperforation
- Check the x-ray for vertebral and radial anomalies
- Do echocardiogram looking for cardiac anomalies
- Do U/S for renal anomalies

Primary surgical repair is preferred, but if it has to be delayed, do a gastrostomy to protect the lungs from acid reflux.

Imperforated anus may be the clinical presentation (noted on physical exam) for the VACTER collection of anomalies. If so, the others have to be ruled out as detailed above.

For the imperforated anus itself, look for a fistula nearby (to vagina or perineum).

- If present, repair can be delayed until further growth (but before toilet training time).
- If not present, do a colostomy for high rectal pouches (and definitive repair at a later date).
  - A primary repair can be done right away if the blind pouch is almost at the anus.
  - The level of the pouch is determined with x-rays taken upside down (so that the gas in the pouch goes up), with a metal marker taped to the anus.

Congenital diaphragmatic hernia is always on the left and results in bowel residing in the chest. The real problem is not the mechanical one, but the hypoplastic lung that still has fetal-type circulation. Repair must be delayed 3–4 days to allow maturation. Babies go into respiratory distress, and need endotracheal intubation, low-pressure ventilation (careful not to hyperinflate the contralateral lung), sedation, and NG suction. Difficult cases may require extracorporeal membrane oxygenation (ECMO). Many patients currently are diagnosed before birth by U/S.

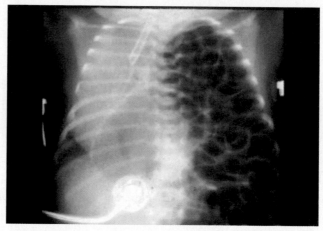

Copyright 2007 Gold Standard Multimedia Inc.

Figure I-5-1. Congenital Diaphragmatic Hernia with Bowel Contents in the Thoracic Cavity

Gastroschisis and omphalocele present with an abdominal wall defect in the abdomen.

- In gastroschisis, the cord is normal (it reaches the baby), the defect is to the right of the cord (lateral), there is no protective membrane, and the bowel looks angry and matted.

- In omphalocele, the cord goes to the defect (central), which has a thin membrane under which one can see a normal-looking bowel and small slice of liver.

Small defects can be closed primarily, but large ones require construction of a Silastic "silo" to house and protect the bowel. The contents of the silo are then squeezed into the belly, a little bit every day, until complete closure can be done in about a week. Babies with gastroschisis also need vascular access for parenteral nutrition, because the angry-looking bowel will not work for about 1 month. If the skin can be closed and not the fascia, then the patient is left with a ventral hernia repaired at a later date.

Exstrophy of the urinary bladder is also an abdominal wall defect, but over the pubis (which is not fused), with a medallion of red bladder mucosa, wet and shining with urine. The baby has to be transferred immediately to a specialized center where a repair can be done within the first 1–2 days of life. Delayed repairs do not work.

Green vomiting in the newborn has ominous significance. A serious problem exists. Green vomiting and a **"double-bubble" picture in x-rays** (a large air-fluid level in the stomach and a smaller one to its right in the first portion of the duodenum) are found in duodenal atresia, annular pancreas, or malrotation. All of these anomalies require surgical correction, but malrotation is the most dangerous because the bowel can twist on itself, cut off its blood supply, and die. If, in addition to the double bubble, there is a little normal gas pattern beyond, the chances of malrotation are higher. Malrotation is diagnosed with contrast enema (safe, but not always diagnostic) or upper GI study (more reliable, but more risky). Although described here as a problem of the newborn, the first signs of malrotation can show up at any time within the first few weeks of life.

Intestinal atresia also shows up with green vomiting, but instead of a double bubble there are multiple air-fluid levels throughout the abdomen. There may be more than one atretic area, but no other congenital anomalies have to be suspected because this condition results from a vascular accident in utero.

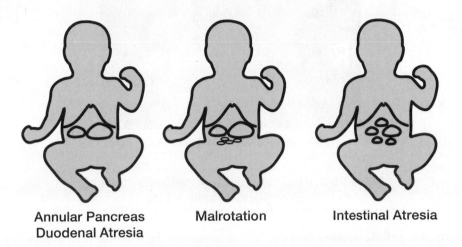

Annular Pancreas   Malrotation   Intestinal Atresia
Duodenal Atresia

A FEW DAYS OLD—FIRST 2 MONTHS OF LIFE

Necrotizing enterocolitis is seen in premature infants when they are first fed. There is feeding intolerance, abdominal distention, and a rapidly dropping platelet count (in babies, a sign of sepsis). Treatment is to stop all feedings and initiate broad-spectrum antibiotics, IV fluids, and nutrition. Surgical intervention is required if they develop abdominal wall erythema, air in the portal vein, intestinal pneumatosis (presence of gas in the bowel wall), or pneumoperitoneum, all signs of intestinal necrosis and perforation.

Meconium ileus is seen in babies who have cystic fibrosis (often hinted at by the mother having it). They develop feeding intolerance and bilious vomiting. X-rays show multiple dilated loops of small bowel and a ground-glass appearance in the lower abdomen. Gastrografin enema is both diagnostic (microcolon and inspissated pellets of meconium in the terminal ileum) and therapeutic (Gastrografin draws fluid in and dissolves the pellets).

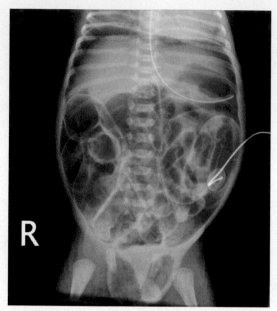

Figure I-5-2. Meconium Ileus with Perforation (Free Air)
seen on Plain Abdominal X-ray

Hypertrophic pyloric stenosis shows up age ~3 weeks, more commonly in first-born boys, with non-bilious projectile vomiting after each feeding. The baby is hungry and eager to eat again after he vomits. By the time they are seen they are dehydrated, with visible gastric peristaltic waves and a palpable "olive-size" mass in the right upper quadrant. If the mass cannot be felt, U/S is diagnostic. Therapy begins with rehydration and correction of the hypochloremic, hypokalemic metabolic alkalosis, followed by pyloromyotomy.

Biliary atresia should be suspected in babies age 6- to 8 weeks who have persistent, progressively increasing jaundice (which includes a substantial conjugated fraction). Do serologies and sweat test to rule out other problems, and do HIDA scan after 1 week of phenobarbital (which is a powerful choleretic). If no bile reaches the duodenum even with phenobarbital stimulation, surgical exploration is needed.

- 1/3 of cases can get a long-lasting surgical derivation
- 1/3 of cases need liver transplant after surviving for a while with a surgical derivation
- 1/3 of cases need transplant right away

Hirschsprung's disease (aganglionic megacolon) can be recognized in early life, or may go undiagnosed for many years. The cardinal symptom is chronic constipation. With short segments, rectal exam may lead to explosive expulsion of stool and flatus, with relief of abdominal distention. In older children in whom differential diagnosis with psychogenic problems is an issue, presence of fecal soiling suggests the latter. X-rays show distended proximal colon (the normal one) and "normal-looking" distal colon, which is the aganglionic part. Diagnosis is made with full-thickness biopsy of rectal mucosa. Ingenious operations have been devised to preserve the unique sensory input of the motor-impaired rectum, while adding the normal propulsive capability of the innervated colon.

LATER IN INFANCY

Intussusception is seen in chubby, healthy looking babies ages 6- to 12 months, who have episodes of colicky abdominal pain which makes them double up and squat. The pain lasts for ~1 minute, and the child looks perfectly happy and normal until he gets another colic episode. Physical exam shows a vague mass on the right side of the abdomen, an "empty" right lower quadrant, and "currant jelly" stools. Barium or air enema is both diagnostic and therapeutic. If reduction is not achieved radiologically (or if there are recurrences), surgery is done.

Child abuse should always be suspected when injuries cannot be properly accounted for. Some classic presentations include:

- Subdural hematoma plus retinal hemorrhages (shaken baby syndrome)
- Multiple fractures in different bones at different stages of healing
- All scalding burns, particularly burns of both buttocks (child was held by arms and legs and dipped into boiling water)

Refer to the proper authorities.

Meckel's diverticulum should be suspected in lower GI bleeding in the pediatric age group. Diagnose with a radioisotope scan looking for gastric mucosa in the lower abdomen.

Cardiothoracic Surgery 6

Learning Objectives

❏ Answer questions about the surgical correction of congenital and acquired heart problems

❏ Describe surgical issues related to diseases of the lung

CONGENITAL HEART PROBLEMS

Vascular ring produces symptoms of pressure on the tracheobronchial tree and pressure on the esophagus.

- The first symptom includes stridor and episodes of respiratory distress with "crowing" respiration, during which the baby assumes a hyperextended position.
- The latter symptoms revolve around some difficulty swallowing. (If only the respiratory symptoms are present, one should think of tracheomalacia.)

Barium swallow shows typical extrinsic compression from the abnormal vessel. Bronchoscopy shows segmental tracheal compression and rules out diffuse tracheomalacia. Surgery divides the smaller of the two aortic arches.

Morphologic cardiac anomalies (congenital or acquired) are best diagnosed with an echocardiogram.

Left-to-right shunts share the presence of a murmur, overloading of the pulmonary circulation, and long-term damage to the pulmonary vasculature. The volume and consequences of the shunt are different at different locations, as noted below.

An **atrial septal defect** has a very minor, low-pressure, low-volume shunt. Patients typically grow into late infancy before they are recognized. A faint pulmonary flow systolic murmur and fixed split second heart sound are characteristic. A history of frequent colds is elicited. Echocardiogram is diagnostic. Closure can be achieved surgically or by cardiac catheterization.

Small, restrictive ventricular septal defects low in the muscular septum produce a heart murmur, but otherwise few symptoms. They are likely to close spontaneously within the first 2 or 3 years of life.

A **ventricular septal defect** (VSD) in the more typical location (high in the membranous septum) leads to trouble early on. Within the first few months there will be "failure to thrive," a loud pansystolic murmur best heard at the left sternal border, and increased pulmonary vascular markings on chest x-ray. Diagnose with an echocardiogram and treat with surgical closure.

Patent ductus arteriosus becomes symptomatic in the first few days of life. There are bounding peripheral pulses and a continuous "machinery-like" heart murmur. Echocardiogram is diagnostic. In premature infants who have not gone into CHF, closure can be achieved with indomethacin. Those which do not close, babies who are in heart failure, or full-term babies need surgical ligation.

Right-to-left shunts share the presence of a murmur, diminished vascular markings in the lung, and cyanosis. Although 5 are always described (all beginning with the letter T), 3 of them are rather rare and will not be reviewed (one of them, truncus arteriosus, is fascinating because it is cyanotic but it kills by overloading the pulmonary circulation, like the noncyanotic shunts do). The common ones follow.

- **Tetralogy of Fallot** (VSD, pulmonary stenosis, overriding aorta, and right ventricular hypertrophy), although crippling, often allows children to grow up into infancy. It is also the most common cyanotic anomaly, and thus any exam question in which a child age 5–6 is cyanotic is bound to be tetralogy. The children are small for their age, have a bluish hue in the lips and tips of their fingers, clubbing, and spells of cyanosis relieved by squatting. There is a systolic ejection murmur in the left third intercostal space, a small heart, diminished pulmonary vascular markings on chest x-ray, and ECG signs of right ventricular hypertrophy. Echocardiogram is diagnostic, treatment is surgical repair.

- **Transposition of the great vessels** leads to severe trouble early on. Children are kept alive by an atrial septal defect, ventricular septal defect, or patent ductus (or a combination), but die very soon if not corrected. Suspect this diagnosis in a child age 1-2 days with cyanosis who is in deep trouble, and ask for echocardiogram. The technical details of the surgical correction are mind-boggling, and you do not have to know them.

ACQUIRED HEART DISEASE

Aortic stenosis produces angina, syncope, and dyspnea. There is a harsh midsystolic heart murmur best heard at the right second intercostal space and along the left sternal border. Start the workup with an echocardiogram. Surgical valvular replacement is indicated if there is a gradient >50 mm Hg, or at the first indication of CHF, angina, or syncope.

Chronic aortic insufficiency produces wide pulse pressure and a blowing, high-pitched, diastolic heart murmur best heard at the second intercostal space and along the left lower sternal border, with the patient in full expiration. Patients are often followed with medical therapy for many years, but should undergo valvular replacement at the first evidence on echocardiogram of the beginning left ventricular dilatation.

Acute aortic insufficiency because of endocarditis is seen in young drug addicts who suddenly develop CHF and a new, loud diastolic murmur at the right second intercostal space. Emergency valve replacement and long-term antibiotics are needed.

Mitral stenosis is caused by a history of rheumatic fever many years before presentation. It produces dyspnea on exertion, orthopnea, paroxysmal nocturnal dyspnea, cough, and hemoptysis. There is a low-pitched, rumbling diastolic apical heart murmur. As it progresses, patients become thin and cachectic and develop atrial fibrillation. Workup starts with echocardiogram. As symptoms become more disabling, mitral valve repair becomes necessary with a surgical commissurotomy or mitral valve replacement.

Mitral regurgitation is most commonly caused by valvular prolapse. Patients develop exertional dyspnea, orthopnea, and atrial fibrillation. There is an apical, high-pitched, holosystolic heart murmur that radiates to the axilla and back. Workup and surgical indications are as above, with repair of the valve (annuloplasty) preferred over prosthetic replacement.

Coronary disease can happen to anybody (including women), but the typical patient is as follows:

- Middle-age sedentary man
- Has family history, smoking history, type II diabetes and/or hypercholesterolemia

Progressive, unstable, disabling angina is the main reason to do cardiac catheterization and evaluate as a potential candidate for revascularization. Intervention is indicated if ≥1 vessels have ≥70% stenosis and there is a good distal vessel. Preferably, the patient should still have good ventricular function (you cannot resuscitate dead myocardium).

The general rule is that the simpler the problem, the more it is amenable to angioplasty and stent; whereas more complex situations do better with surgery.

- Single vessel disease (that is not the left main or the anterior descending) is perfect for angioplasty and stent.
- Triple vessel disease makes multiple coronary bypass (using the internal mammary for the most important vessel) the best choice.

Post-operative care of heart surgery patients often requires that cardiac output be optimized. If cardiac output is considerably under normal (5 liters/min, or cardiac index 3), the pulmonary wedge pressure (or left atrial pressure, or left end-diastolic pressure) should be measured. Low numbers (0–3) suggest the need for more IV fluids. High numbers (≥20) suggest ventricular failure.

Chronic constrictive pericarditis produces dyspnea on exertion, hepatomegaly, and ascites, and shows a classic "square root sign" and equalization of pressures (right atrial, right ventricular diastolic, pulmonary artery diastolic, pulmonary capillary wedge, and left ventricular diastolic) on cardiac catheterization. Surgical therapy relieves it.

LUNG

A **solitary "coin" lesion** found on a chest x-ray has an 80% chance of being malignant in people age >50, and even higher if there is a significant history of smoking. A very expensive workup for cancer of the lung, however, can be avoided if an older chest x-ray shows the same unchanged lesion; it is unlikely to be cancer. Therefore, seeking an older x-ray is always the first step when a solitary pulmonary nodule is detected.

Suspected **cancer of the lung** requires what is potentially an expensive and invasive workup to confirm diagnosis and assess operability. It starts with a chest x-ray (which may have been ordered because of persistent cough or hemoptysis) showing a suspicious lesion. Assuming no older x-ray is available or the lesion was not present on a previous film, 2 noninvasive tests should be done first: sputum cytology and CT scan (chest and upper abdomen).

Diagnosis of cancer of the lung, if not established by cytology, requires bronchoscopy and biopsies (for central lesions) or percutaneous biopsy (for peripheral lesions). If unsuccessful with those, video-assisted thoracic surgery (VATS) and wedge resection may be needed. How far one goes in that sequence depends on the following:

- Probability of cancer (higher in elderly, with history of smoking and noncalcified lesion in CT)
- Assurance that surgery can be done (residual pulmonary function will suffice)
- Chances that the surgery may be curative (no metastases to mediastinal or carinal nodes, the other lung, or the liver)

The interplay of these factors determines the specific sequence of workup beyond sputum cytology and CT scan in each patient.

Small cell cancer of the lung is treated with chemotherapy and radiation, and therefore assessment of operability and curative chances of surgery are not applicable. Operability and possibility of surgical cure applies only to non–small cell cancer.

The operability of lung cancer is predicated on residual function after resection. If clinical findings (COPD, shortness of breath) suggest this may be the limiting factor, do pulmonary function studies.

- Determine FEV1
- Determine fraction that comes from each lung (by ventilation-perfusion scan)
- Figure out what would remain after pneumonectomy

A minimum FEV_1 of 800 mL is mandatory for a patient to undergo lung resection, as the worst case scenario is that a pneumonectomy will need to be performed and could potentially leave a marginal patient ventilator dependent. If <800 mL, do not continue expensive tests; the patient is not a surgical candidate. Treat with chemotherapy and radiation instead.

Potential cure by surgical removal of lung cancer depends on extent of metastases.

- Hilar metastases can be removed with the pneumonectomy.
- Nodal metastases at the carina or mediastinum preclude curative resection.
- CT scan may identify nodal metastases.
- The addition of PET scan has helped define the presence of an actively growing tumor in enlarged nodes.
- Endobronchial U/S has emerged as a mainstay of diagnosis by obtaining tissue samples from mediastinal nodes; cervical mediastinal exploration ("mediastinoscopy") is now rarely needed.
- Metastases to the contralateral lung, adrenal gland, or liver would also be evident in the CT and be a contraindication to surgical resection.

Vascular Surgery 7

Learning Objectives

❑ List the common procedures, including indications, complications, and alternatives, in vascular surgery

Subclavian steal syndrome is rare but fascinating (medical school professors love it, thus it is likely to appear on exams). An arteriosclerotic stenotic plaque at the origin of the subclavian (proximal to the takeoff of the vertebral) allows enough blood supply to reach the arm for normal activity, but does not allow enough to meet higher demands when the arm is exercised. When that happens, the arm sucks blood away from the brain by reversing the flow in the vertebral.

Clinically the patient describes claudication of the arm (coldness, tingling, muscle pain) and posterior neurologic signs (visual symptoms, equilibrium problems) when the arm is exercised. Vascular symptoms alone would suggest thoracic outlet syndrome, but the combination with neurologic symptoms identifies the subclavian steal. Duplex scanning is diagnostic when it shows reversal of flow. Bypass surgery is curative.

Abdominal aortic aneurysm (AAA) is typically asymptomatic, found as a pulsatile abdominal mass on examination (between the xiphoid and the umbilicus), or found on x-rays, U/S, or CT scans done for another diagnostic purpose, usually in an older man. Size is the key to management; if an aneurysm is found by physical exam, U/S or CT scan is needed to provide precise measurements.

- If aneurysm is ≤4 cm, it can be safely observed; chance of rupture is almost zero
- If aneurysm is ≥5 cm, patient should have elective repair because chance of rupture is very high

Aneurysms that grow 1 cm per year or faster also need elective repair. Most AAAs are now treated with endovascular stents inserted percutaneously. The 10-year outcome has been encouraging; limiting factors to this modality are specific anatomic criteria (neck of aneurysm, landing zone, and tortuosity of vascular tree) and available resources (angiography team and equipment). Open AAA repair involves an interposition graft within the aneurysm sac and carries ~10-15% peri-operative morbidity, with MI, renal failure, and bowel ischemia being the most severe culprits.

Surgery for a ruptured AAA carries very high morbidity and mortality, thus efforts are made to predict and anticipate rupture, and not wait for it to occur.

- A tender AAA is at risk to rupture, so immediate repair is indicated.
- Excruciating back pain in a patient with a large AAA means that the aneurysm is already leaking. Retroperitoneal hematoma is already forming, and blowout into the peritoneal cavity is imminent; emergency surgery is required.

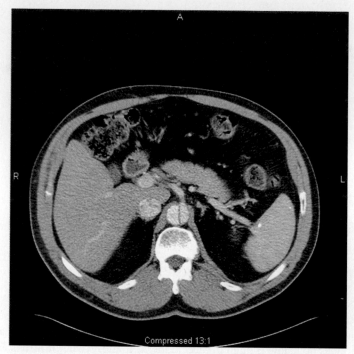

Figure I-7-1. CT Scan of 52-year-old Man with an
Abdominal Aortic Aneurysm Involving the Celiac Artery

Arteriosclerotic occlusive disease of the lower extremities has an unpredictable natural history (except for the predictable negative impact of smoking), and therefore there is no role for "prophylactic" surgery in claudication. Surgery is done only to relieve disabling symptoms or to save the extremity from impending necrosis (rest pain). The first clinical manifestation is pain brought about by walking and relieved by rest (intermittent claudication). If the claudication does not interfere significantly with the patient's lifestyle, no workup is indicated. Smoking cessation, exercise, and the use of cilostazol can help the patient in the long run.

The workup of **disabling intermittent claudication** starts with Doppler studies looking for a pressure gradient.

- If there isn't a significant gradient, the disease is in the small vessels and not amenable to surgery. If there is one, CTA or magnetic resonance angiogram is performed to identify specific areas of stenosis or complete obstruction, and to look for good distal vessels to which a bypass graft could be anastomosed.

- Short stenotic segments can be treated with angioplasty and stenting.

- More extensive disease may require bypass grafts, sequential stents or longer stents.

- When multiple lesions are present, proximal ones are usually repaired before distal ones are addressed.

- Grafts originating at the aorta (aortobifemoral) are done with prosthetic material.

- Bypasses between more distal vessels (femoropopliteal, or beyond) are usually done with reversed saphenous vein grafts.

Rest pain is the penultimate stage of the disease (the ultimate is ulceration and gangrene). The clinical picture is rather characteristic. The patient seeks help because he "cannot sleep." It turns out that pain in the calf is what keeps him from falling asleep. He has learned that sitting up and dangling the leg helps the pain, and a few minutes after he does so, the leg that used to be very pale becomes deep purple. Physical exam shows shiny atrophic skin without hair, and no peripheral pulses. Workup and therapy are as detailed above.

Arterial embolization from a distant source is seen in patients with atrial fibrillation (a clot breaks off from the atrial appendage) or those with a recent MI (the source of the embolus is the mural thrombus). The patient suddenly develops the 6 Ps:

- Painful
- Pale
- Cold ("poikilothermic")
- Pulseless
- Paresthetic
- Paralytic lower extremity

Urgent evaluation and treatment should be completed within 6 hours. Doppler studies will locate the point of obstruction. Early incomplete occlusion may be treated with clot busters. Embolectomy with Fogarty catheters is effective for complete obstructions, and fasciotomy should be added if several hours have passed before revascularization to prevent compartment syndrome from reperfusion edema.

Dissecting aneurysm of the thoracic aorta occurs in the poorly controlled hypertensive. The episode resembles an MI, with sudden onset of extremely severe, tearing chest pain that radiates to the back and migrates down shortly after its onset. There may be unequal pulses in the upper extremities, and chest x-ray shows a widened mediastinum. ECG and cardiac enzymes rule out an MI. Definitive diagnosis should be sought by noninvasive means such as CTA or MRA, but TEE is useful as well. Type A dissections (involving the ascending aorta) are treated surgically, whereas Type B (those in the descending only) are managed medically with control of the hypertension in the ICU.

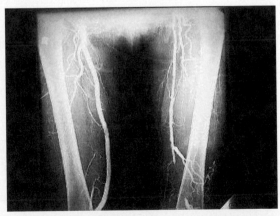

Copyright 2007 Gold Standard Multimedia Inc.

Figure I-7-2. Peripheral Vascular Disease noted on Angiogram of the Lower Extremities

Skin Surgery 8

Learning Objectives

❏ List the common procedures, including indications, complications, and alternatives, in dermatology

Cancer of the skin is typically seen in blond, blue-eyed, fair-skinned people who live where the sun is fierce, and who by virtue of occupation or hobby are out in the sun all day.

- Basal cell carcinoma: 50% of cases
- Squamous cell carcinoma: 25% of cases
- Melanoma: ≥15% of cases (incidence is rising)

They have preferred presentations (detailed below), but diagnosis in all is done by obtaining tissue from a biopsy of the lesion (shave, punch or excisional biopsy). Excisional biopsy is the most accurate in diagnosis, especially when melanoma is suspected. Because they share etiology, they often coexist, and patients frequently have multiple lesions over the years.

Basal cell carcinoma may show up as a raised waxy lesion or as a nonhealing ulcer. It has a preference for the upper part of the face (above a line drawn across the lips). It does not metastasize, but can kill by relentless local invasion ("rodent ulcer"). Local excision with negative margins (1 mm is enough) is curative, but other lesions may develop later.

Squamous cell carcinoma of the skin shows up as a nonhealing ulcer, has a preference for the lower lip (and territories below a line drawn across the lips), and can metastasize to lymph nodes. Excision with wider margins is needed (0.5–2 cm), and node dissection is done if they are involved. Radiation treatment is another option.

Melanoma usually originates in a pigmented lesion. A mnemonic to identify them is **ABCD**.

- Asymmetric (A)
- Irregular borders (B)
- Different colors (C) within the lesion
- Diameter (D) >0.5 cm

Melanoma should also be suspected in any pigmented lesion that changes in any way (grows, ulcerates, changes color and/or shape, bleeds, etc.). The biopsy report must give not only the diagnosis, but also the depth of invasion. The prognosis of melanoma is directly related to the thickness or depth of invasion (Breslow measurement); the deeper the thickness/depth of invasion, the worse the prognosis.

Table I-8-1. Breslow Measurements

Thickness/Depth	Surgical Margins Required
MIS (melanoma in-situ)	0.5 cm
<1 mm	1 cm
1-2 mm	1-2 cm
>2 mm	2 cm

Melanoma-in-situ (non-invasive melanoma) carries an excellent prognosis and can be effectively treated with local excison (5 mm margins).

- Lesions <1 mm in depth have a good prognosis and require only local excision with 1 cm margins.

- Lesions 1–2 cm in depth have a worse prognosis and require resection with 1-2 cm margins.

- Deeper lesions (>2 mm) require excision with wide margins (2 cm).

- Lesions >4 mm have a poor prognosis.

- Lesions 1–4 mm benefit most from aggressive therapy, including management of nodes.

- Patients with lesions >1 mm deep and without palpable nodes on exam should undergo sentinel lymph node biopsy.

Metastatic malignant melanoma (from a deep, invasive primary) can be aggressive and unpredictable. Melanoma can metastasize to all the usual places (lymph nodes, liver, lung, brain, and bone), but it can also metastasize to remote and bizarre locations (e.g. the muscle of the left ventricle, the wall of the duodenum…anywhere!).

Furthermore, it has no predictable timetable. Some patients are full of metastases within a few months of diagnosis, while others go 20 years between resection of their primary tumor and the sudden explosion of metastases. Interferon alpha and ipilimumab are standard options for adjuvant therapy for high-risk melanoma. Newer drugs such as Anti-PD-1 Antibodies are being explored for treatment.

Ophthalmology 9

Learning Objectives

❏ List the common procedures, including indications, complications, and alternatives, in ophthalmology

CHILDREN

Amblyopia is a vision impairment caused by interference with the processing of images by the brain during the first 6 or 7 years of life. The most common expression of this phenomenon is the child with strabismus. Faced with two overlapping images, the brain suppresses one of them. If the strabismus is not corrected early on, there will be permanent cortical blindness of the suppressed eye, even though the eye is perfectly normal. Should an obstacle impede vision in one eye during those early years (for instance, a congenital cataract), the same problem will develop.

Strabismus is verified by showing that the reflection from a light comes from different areas of the cornea in each eye. Strabismus should be surgically corrected when diagnosed, to prevent the development of amblyopia. When reliable parents relate that a child did not have strabismus in the early years but develops it later in infancy, the problem is an exaggerated convergence caused by refraction difficulties. In that case corrective glasses instantly resolve the problem. True strabismus does not resolve spontaneously.

A **white pupil in a baby** is an ophthalmologic emergency, as it may be caused by a retinoblastoma. Even if the white pupil is caused by a less lethal problem, like a congenital cataract, it should be attended to in order to prevent amblyopia.

ADULTS

Glaucoma is a very common source of blindness, but because of its silent nature is unlikely to be discovered by regular physicians (or to be tested for in an exam). One variant, however, should be recognized by every physician who might encounter it. **Acute closed angle glaucoma** shows up as very severe eye pain or frontal headache, typically starting in the evening when the pupils have been dilated for several hours (watching a double feature at the movies, or watching television in a dark room).

- Patient may report seeing halos around lights
- On physical exam the pupil is mid-dilated and does not react to light; cornea is cloudy with greenish hue; and eye feels "hard as a rock"

- Emergency treatment is required (ophthalmologists will drill a hole in the iris with a laser beam to provide a drainage route for the fluid that is trapped in the anterior chamber).
- While waiting for the ophthalmologist, administer systemic carbonic anhydrase inhibitors (such as Diamox) and apply topical beta-blockers and alpha-2–selective adrenergic agonists. Mannitol and pilocarpine may also be used.

Orbital cellulitis is another ophthalmologic emergency. The eyelids are hot, tender, red, and swollen; and the patient is febrile—but the key finding when the eyelids are pried open is that the pupil is dilated and fixed, and the eye has very limited motion. There is pus in the orbit, and emergency CT scan and drainage have to be done.

Chemical burns of the eye require massive irrigation, like their counterparts elsewhere in the body. Start irrigation with plain water as soon as possible, and do not wait until arrival at the hospital. Once the eye has been pried open and washed under running water for about 30 minutes, get the patient to the ED. At the hospital, irrigation with saline is continued, corrosive particles are removed from hidden corners, and before the patient is sent home, pH is tested to assure that no harmful chemicals remain in the conjunctival sac. As is true elsewhere in the body, alkaline burns are worse than acid burns.

Retinal detachment is another emergency that should be recognized by all physicians. The patient reports seeing flashes of light and having "floaters" in the eye. The number of floaters gives a rough idea of the magnitude of the problem.

- The person with 1 or 2 floaters may only have vitreous tugging at the retina, with little actual detachment.
- The person who describes dozens of floaters, or "a snow storm" within the eye, or a big dark cloud at the top of his visual field has a big horseshoe piece of the retina pulled away, and is at risk of ripping out the rest. Emergency intervention, with laser "spot welding," will protect the remaining retina.

Embolic occlusion of the retinal artery is also an emergency, although little can be done about it. The patient (typically elderly) describes sudden loss of vision from one eye. In about 30 minutes the damage will be irreversible, but the standard recommendation is for the patient to breathe into a paper bag, and have someone repeatedly press hard on the eye and release while he is in transit to the ED (the idea is to vasodilate and shake the clot into a more distal location, so that a smaller area is ischemic).

Newly diagnosed diabetics need ophthalmologic evaluation if they have type II, because they may have had it for years before diagnosis was made. Retinal damage may have already occurred, and proper treatment may prevent its progression. Young people diagnosed with type I are about 20 years away from getting eye problems.

10

Learning Objectives

❑ List the most important ENT emergencies and describe the presenting features of each

❑ Describe the common neck masses and ENT tumors including prognosis

❑ Recognize and present treatment options for pediatric ENT problems

NECK MASSES

Neck masses can be congenital, inflammatory, or neoplastic. Congenital masses are seen in young people, and typically have been present for years before they become symptomatic (get infected) and medical help is sought. The timetable of inflammatory masses is typically measured in days or weeks. After a few weeks an inflammatory mass has reached some kind of resolution (drained or resolved). The timetable of neoplastic masses is typically several months of relentless growth.

Congenital

Thyroglossal duct cyst is located on the midline, at the level of the hyoid bone, and originates from the foramen cecum in the tongue (pulling at the tongue retracts the mass). It is typically 1–2 cm in diameter. Surgical removal includes the cyst, the middle segment of the hyoid bone, and the track that leads to the base of the tongue (Sistrunk procedure).

Branchial cleft cyst occurs laterally, along the anterior edge of the sternomastoid muscle, anywhere from in front of the tragus to the base of the neck. It is typically several centimeters in diameter, and sometimes has a little opening and blind tract in the skin overlying it.

Cystic hygroma is found at the base of the neck as a large, mushy, ill-defined mass that occupies the entire supraclavicular area and seems to extend deeper into the chest. Indeed, it often extends into the mediastinum, and therefore CT scan before attempted surgical removal is mandatory.

Inflammatory versus Neoplastic

Most recently discovered enlarged lymph nodes are benign, and so an extensive workup should not be undertaken right away. Complete history and physical should be followed by an appointment in 3 to 4 weeks. If the mass is still there, workup then follows.

Persistent enlarged lymph node (a history of weeks or months) could still be inflammatory, but neoplasia has to be ruled out. There are several patterns that are suggestive of specific diagnosis, as detailed below.

Lymphoma is typically seen in young people; they often have multiple enlarged nodes (in the neck and elsewhere) and have been suffering from low-grade fever and night sweats. FNA can be done, but usually a node has to be removed for pathologic study to determine specific type. Chemotherapy is the usual treatment.

Metastatic tumor to supraclavicular nodes invariably comes from below the clavicles (and not from the head and neck). Lung or intraabdominal tumors are the usual primaries. The node itself may be removed to help establish a tissue diagnosis. It is commonly on the left side (Virchow's node).

Squamous cell carcinoma of the mucosae of the head and neck is seen in older men who smoke, drink, and have rotten teeth. Patients with AIDS are also prime candidates. Often the first manifestation is a metastatic node in the neck (typically to the jugular chain). The ideal diagnostic workup is a triple endoscopy (or panendoscopy) looking for the primary tumor.

- Biopsy of the primary establishes the diagnosis, and CT scan demonstrates the extent.
- FNA of the node may be done, but open biopsy of the neck mass should never be performed, as an incision in the neck will eventually interfere with the appropriate surgical approach for the tumor.

Treatment involves resection, radical neck dissection, and very often radiotherapy and platinum-based chemotherapy. Other presentations of squamous cell carcinoma include persistent hoarseness, persistent painless ulcer in the floor of the mouth, and persistent unilateral earache.

OTHER TUMORS

Acoustic nerve neuroma should be suspected in an adult who has sensory hearing loss in one ear, but not the other (and who does not engage in sport shooting that would subject one ear to more noise than the other). MRI is the best diagnostic modality.

Facial nerve tumors produce gradual unilateral facial nerve paralysis affecting both the forehead and the lower face, as opposed to sudden onset paralysis which suggests Bell's palsy. Gadolinium-enhanced MRI is the best diagnostic study.

Parotid tumors are visible and palpable in front of the ear, or around the angle of the mandible. Most are pleomorphic adenomas, which are benign but have potential for malignant degeneration. They do not produce pain or facial nerve paralysis. A hard parotid mass that is painful or has produced paralysis is a parotid cancer.

- FNA of these tumors may be done, but open biopsy is absolutely contraindicated.
- A formal superficial parotidectomy (or superficial and deep if the tumor is deep to the facial nerve) is the appropriate way to excise—and thereby biopsy—parotid tumors, preventing recurrences and sparing the facial nerve.
- Enucleation alone leads to recurrence.
- In malignant tumors the nerve is sacrificed and a nerve interposition graft performed.

PEDIATRIC ENT

Foreign bodies are the cause of unilateral ENT problems in toddlers. A 2-year-old with unilateral earache, unilateral rhinorrhea, or unilateral wheezing has a little toy truck (or another small toy) in his ear canal, up his nose, or into a bronchus. The appropriate endoscopy under anesthesia will allow extraction.

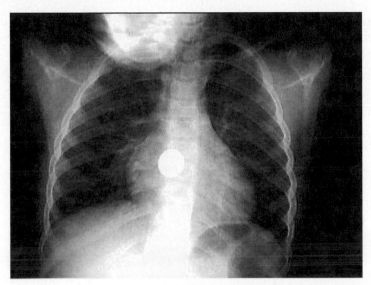

Copyright 2007 Gold Standard Multimedia Inc.

Figure I-10-1. Airway Foreign Body Noted on Chest X-ray

ENT EMERGENCIES AND MISCELLANEOUS

Ludwig's angina is an abscess of the floor of the mouth, often the result of a bad tooth infection. The usual findings of an abscess are present, but the special issue here is the threat to the airway. Incision and drainage are done, but intubation and tracheostomy may also be needed to protect the airway.

Bell's palsy produces sudden paralysis of the facial nerve for no apparent reason. Although not an emergency per se, current practice includes the use of antiviral medications—and as is the case for other situations in which antivirals are used, prompt and early administration is the key to their success. Steroids are also typically prescribed.

Facial nerve injuries sustained in multiple trauma produce paralysis right away. Patients who have normal nerve function at the time of admission and later develop paralysis have swelling that will resolve spontaneously.

Cavernous sinus thrombosis is heralded by the development of diplopia (from paralysis of extrinsic eye muscles) in a patient suffering from frontal or ethmoid sinusitis. This is a serious emergency that requires hospitalization, IV antibiotics, CT scans, and drainage of the affected sinuses.

Epistaxis in children is typically from nosepicking; the bleeding comes from the anterior septum, and phenylephrine spray and local pressure controls the problem. In teenagers the prime suspects are cocaine abuse (with septal perforation) or juvenile nasopharyngeal angiofibroma. Posterior packing may be needed for the former, and surgical resection is mandatory for the latter (the tumor is benign, but it eats away at nearby structures).

In the elderly and hypertensive, nosebleeds can be copious and life-threatening. BP has to be controlled, and posterior packing is usually required. Sometimes angiographic or surgical ligation of feeding vessels is the only way to control the problem.

Dizziness may be caused by inner ear disease or cerebral disease. When the inner ear is the culprit, the patients describe the room spinning around them (vertigo). When the problem is in the brain, the patient is unsteady but the room is perceived to be stable. In the first case meclizine, Phenergan, or diazepam may help. In the second case, neurologic workup is in order.

Neurosurgery 11

Learning Objectives

❏ List differential diagnoses for neurosurgical presenting complaints

❏ Describe neurosurgical treatment options for cerebrovascular occlusive disease

❏ Describe primary and metastatic brain tumors, treatment options, and prognosis

❏ Provide an approach to treating chronic pain syndromes

DIFFERENTIAL DIAGNOSIS BASED ON PATIENT HISTORY

The timetable and mode of presentation of neurologic disease may provide the first clues as to its nature.

- **Vascular problems** have sudden onset without headache when they are occlusive, and with very severe headache when they are hemorrhagic.

- **Brain tumors** have a timetable of months, and produce constant, progressive, severe headache, sometimes worse in the mornings. As intracranial pressure increases, blurred vision and projectile vomiting are added. If the tumor presses on an area of the brain associated with a particular function, deficits of that function may be evident.

- **Infectious problems** have a timetable of days or weeks, and often an identifiable source of infection in the history.

- **Metabolic problems** develop rapidly (hours or days) and affect the entire CNS. Degenerative diseases usually have a timetable of years.

VASCULAR OCCLUSIVE DISEASE

Transient ischemic attack (TIA) is sudden, transitory loss of neurologic function that comes on without headache and resolves spontaneously within 24 hours, leaving no neurologic sequelae. The specific symptoms depend on the area of the brain affected, which is in turn related to the vessels involved. The most common origin is high-grade stenosis (≥70%) of the internal carotid, or ulcerated plaque at the carotid bifurcation.

- The importance of TIAs is that they are predictors of stroke, and timely elective carotid endarterectomy may prevent or minimize that possibility.

- Workup starts with noninvasive Duplex studies.

- Carotid endarterectomy is indicated if the lesions are found in the location that explains the neurologic symptoms.

- Angioplasty and stent can be performed in high risk surgical patients.

Ischemic stroke also has sudden onset without headache, but the neurologic deficits are present >24 hours, leaving permanent sequelae. Except for very early strokes, ischemic stroke is no longer amenable to revascularization procedures. An ischemic infarct may be complicated by a hemorrhagic infarct if blood supply to the brain is suddenly increased. Vascular workup will eventually be done to identify lesions that might produce another stroke (and treat them), but for the existing infarct, assessment is by CT scan, and therapy is centered on rehabilitation.

There is a current movement to reeducate physicians to recognize very early stroke and treat it emergently with clot busters. CT scan is done first to rule out extensive infarcts or the presence of hemorrhage. IV infusion of tissue-type plasminogen activator (t-PA) is best if started within 90 minutes up to 3 hours after the onset of symptoms.

Intracranial Bleeding

Hemorrhagic stroke is seen in the uncontrolled hypertensive who complains of very severe headache of sudden onset and goes on to develop severe neurologic deficits. CT scan is used to evaluate the location and extent of the hemorrhage, and therapy is directed at control of the hypertension and rehabilitation efforts.

Subarachnoid hemorrhage can be caused by rupture of an intracranial aneurysm as well as trauma or even spontaneous bleeding. The amount of pressure the free blood exerts on the brain determines the severity of symptoms and thereby outcome.

- With **significant pressure exertion**, especially when caused by an aneurysm, patients complain of severe, sudden onset headache—"the worst of their life." Physical exam can demonstrate nuchal rigidity due to meningeal irritation. Evaluation begins with CT scan and may require magnetic resonance angiogram (MRA) or formal angiogram to delineate the neurovascular anatomy. Treatment is either open clipping of the aneurysm or endovascular coiling with good results.
- With **minimal pressure exertion** on the brain, patients are not very symptomatic and do not necessarily seek medical attention or are not fully evaluated; they tend to re-present in a delayed fashion, usually 7-10 days after the "sentinel bleed." When this happens, the degree of intracranial hematoma is often significant, and patients are not always salvageable. Accordingly, a very high index of suspicion at initial presentation can be life-saving.

BRAIN TUMOR

Brain tumor may offer no clue as to location if it presses on a "silent area" of the brain. The only history will be progressively increasing headache for several months, worse in the mornings, and eventually accompanied by signs of increased intracranial pressure:

- Blurred vision
- Papilledema
- Projectile vomiting
- Bradycardia and hypertension (due to Cushing reflex) at the extreme end of the spectrum

Brain tumor can be visualized very well on CT scan, but MRI gives better detail and is the preferred study. While awaiting surgical removal, treat any increased intracranial pressure with high-dose steroids (i.e., dexamethasone).

Clinical localization of brain tumors may be possible by virtue of specific neurologic deficits or symptom patterns. For example, the motor strip and speech centers are often affected in tumors that press on the lateral side of the brain, producing symptoms on the opposite side of the body (people speak with the same side of the brain that controls their dominant hand). Other classic clinical pictures include the following:

- **Tumor at the base of the frontal lobe** produces inappropriate behavior, optic nerve atrophy on the side of the tumor, papilledema on the other side, and anosmia (Foster-Kennedy syndrome).

- **Craniopharyngioma** occurs in children who are short for their age, and they show bitemporal hemianopsia and a calcified lesion above the sella on x-rays.

- **Prolactinomas** produce amenorrhea and galactorrhea in young women. Diagnostic workup includes ruling out pregnancy (pregnancy test), ruling out hypothyroidism, determination of prolactin level, and MRI of the sella. Therapy is with bromocriptine. Transnasal, trans-sphenoidal surgical removal is reserved for those who wish to get pregnant, or those who fail to respond to bromocriptine.

- **Acromegaly** is recognized by the huge hands, feet, tongue, and jaws. (On the exam, images typically show both hands on either side of the face in a frontal view, and a long prominent jaw in a lateral view.) Additionally, there is hypertension, diabetes, sweaty hands, headache, and the history of wedding bands or hats that no longer fit. Workup starts with determination of somatomedin C, and pituitary MRI. Surgical removal is preferred, but radiation is an option.

- **Pituitary apoplexy** occurs when there is bleeding into a pituitary tumor, with subsequent destruction of the pituitary gland. The history may have clues to the long-standing presence of the pituitary tumor (headache, visual loss, endocrine problems), and the acute episode starts with a severe headache, followed by signs of increased compression of nearby structures by the hematoma (deterioration of remaining vision, bilateral pallor of the optic nerves) and pituitary destruction (stupor and hypotension). Steroid replacement is urgently needed, and eventually other hormones will need to be replaced. MRI or CT scan will show the extent of the problem.

- **Tumor of the pineal gland** produces loss of upper gaze and the physical finding known as "sunset eyes" (Parinaud syndrome).

- **Brain tumor in children** is most commonly in the posterior fossa. It produces cerebellar symptoms (stumbling around, truncal ataxia) and the children often assume the knee-chest position to relieve their headache.

- **Brain abscess** shows many of the same manifestations of brain tumors (it is a space-occupying lesion), but much more quickly (a week or two). There is fever, and usually an obvious source of the infection nearby, like otitis media and mastoiditis. It has a very typical appearance on CT, thus the more expensive MRI is not needed. Actual resection is required.

PAIN SYNDROMES

Trigeminal neuralgia (tic douloureux) produces extremely severe, sharp shooting pain in the face, "like a bolt of lightning" brought about by touching a specific area, and lasting about 60 seconds. Patients are in their sixties, and have a completely normal neurologic exam. The only finding on physical exam may be an unshaven area in the face (the trigger zone, which the patient avoids touching). MRI is done to rule out organic lesions. Treatment with anticonvulsants is often successful. If not, radiofrequency ablation can be done.

Reflex sympathetic dystrophy (causalgia) develops several months after a crushing injury. There is constant, burning, agonizing pain that does not respond to the usual analgesics. The pain is aggravated by the slightest stimulation of the area. The extremity is cold, cyanotic, and moist. A successful sympathetic block is diagnostic, and surgical sympathectomy is curative.

Urology 12

Learning Objectives

❏ Describe treatment options for urologic emergencies, including stones and retention

❏ List common congenital urologic diseases and their treatment

❏ Answer questions about urological tumor

❏ Outline the causes and treatments of urinary incontinence

UROLOGIC EMERGENCIES

Testicular torsion is seen in young adolescents. There is severe testicular pain of sudden onset, but no fever, pyuria, or history of recent mumps. The testis is swollen, exquisitely tender, "high riding," and with a "horizontal lie." The cord is not tender. This is one of the few urologic emergencies, and time wasted doing any tests is tantamount to malpractice. Immediate surgical intervention is indicated. After the testis is untwisted, an orchiopexy is done to prevent recurrence; simultaneous contralateral orchiopexy is also indicated.

Acute epididymitis can be confused with testicular torsion. It is seen in young men old enough to be sexually active, and it also starts with severe testicular pain of sudden onset. There is fever and pyuria, and although the testis is swollen and very tender, is in the normal position. The cord is also very tender. Acute epididymitis is treated with antibiotics, but the possibility of missing a diagnosis of testicular torsion is so dreadful that sonogram is done to rule it out.

The combination of **obstruction and infection of the urinary tract** is the other condition (besides testicular torsion) that is a dire emergency. Any situation in which these two conditions coexist can lead to destruction of the kidney in a few hours, and potentially to death from sepsis. A typical scenario is a patient who is being allowed to pass a ureteral stone spontaneously, and who suddenly develops chills, fever spike (104–105°F), and flank pain. In addition to IV antibiotics, immediate decompression of the urinary tract above the obstruction is required. This is accomplished by the quickest and simplest means (in this example, ureteral stent or percutaneous nephrostomy), deferring more elaborate instrumentations for a later, safer date.

UTI (cystitis) is very common in women of reproductive age and requires no elaborate workup. Patients have frequency, painful urination, with small volumes of cloudy and malodorous urine. Empiric antimicrobial therapy is used. More serious infection such as pyelonephritis, or UTI in children or young men, requires urinary cultures and a urologic workup to rule out concomitant obstruction as the reason for the serious infection.

Pyelonephritis produces chills, high fever, nausea and vomiting, and flank pain. Hospitalization, IV antibiotics (guided by cultures), and urologic workup (IVP or sonogram) are required.

Acute bacterial prostatitis is seen in older men who have chills, fever, dysuria, urinary frequency, diffuse low back pain, and an exquisitely tender prostate on rectal exam. IV antibiotics are indicated, and care should be taken not to repeat any more rectal exams. Continued prostatic massage could lead to septic shock.

CONGENITAL UROLOGIC DISEASE

Posterior urethral valve is the most common reason a newborn boy doesn't urinate during day 1 of life (also look for meatal stenosis). Gentle catheterization can be done to empty the bladder (the valves will not present an obstacle to the catheter). Voiding cystourethrogram is the diagnostic test, and endoscopic fulguration or resection will get rid of them.

Hypospadias is easily noted on physical exam. The urethral opening is on the ventral side of the penis, somewhere between the tip and the base of the shaft. Circumcision should never be done on such a child, inasmuch as the skin of the prepuce will be needed for the plastic reconstruction that will eventually be done.

UTI in children should always lead to a urologic workup. The cause may be vesicoureteral reflux, or some other congenital anomaly. **Vesicoureteral reflux** and infection produce burning on urination, frequency, low abdominal and perineal pain, flank pain, and fever and chills in a child. Start treatment of the infection (empiric antibiotics first, followed by culture-guided choice), and do IVP and voiding cystogram looking for the reflux. If found, use long-term antibiotics until the child "grows out of the problem."

Low implantation of a ureter is usually asymptomatic in little boys but has a fascinating clinical presentation in little girls. The patient feels normally the need to void, and voids normally at appropriate intervals (urine deposited into the bladder by the normal ureter); but is also wet with urine all the time (urine that drips into the vagina from the low implanted ureter). If physical examination does not find the abnormal ureteral opening, IVP will show it. Corrective surgery is done.

Ureteropelvic junction (UPJ) obstruction can also produce a fascinating clinical presentation. The anomaly at the UPJ allows normal urinary output to flow without difficulty, but if a large diuresis occurs, the narrow area cannot handle it. Thus the classic presentation is an adolescent who goes on a beer-drinking binge for the first time in his life, and develops colicky flank pain.

TUMORS

Hematuria is the most common presentation for cancers of the kidney, ureter, or bladder. Actually most cases of hematuria are caused by benign disease, but except for the adult who has a trace of urine after significant trauma, any patient presenting with hematuria needs a workup to rule out cancer. Workup should begin with CT scan and continue with cystoscopy, which is the only reliable way to rule out cancer of the bladder.

Renal cell carcinoma in its full-blown picture produces hematuria, flank pain, and a flank mass. It can also produce hypercalcemia, erythrocytosis, and elevated liver enzymes. That full-blown picture is rarely seen today, since most patients are worked up as soon as they have hematuria. CT gives the best detail, showing the mass to be a heterogenic solid tumor (and alerting the urologist to potential growth into the renal vein and the vena cava). Surgery is the only effective therapy and may include partial nephrectomy, radical nephrectomy, or even inferior vena cava resection.

Cancer of the bladder (transitional cell cancer in most cases) has a very close correlation with smoking (even more so than cancer of the lung), and usually presents with hematuria. Sometimes there are irritative voiding symptoms, and patients may have been treated for UTI even though cultures were negative and they were afebrile. Although cystoscopy is the best way to diagnose these, it should be preceded by CT scan. Both surgery and intravesical BCG have therapeutic roles, and a very high rate of local recurrence makes life-long close follow-up a necessity.

Prostatic cancer incidence increases with age. Most are asymptomatic, and have to be sought by rectal exam (rock-hard discrete nodule) and prostatic specific antigen (PSA; elevated levels for age group). Surveillance frequently stops at age 75, beyond which survival is not affected by treatment. Transrectal needle biopsy (guided by sonogram when discovered by PSA) establishes diagnosis. CT helps assess extent and type of therapy. Surgery and/or radiation are choices. Widespread bone metastases respond for a few years to androgen ablation, surgical (orchiectomy) or medical (luteinizing hormone-releasing hormone agonists or antiandrogens like flutamide).

Testicular cancer affects young men, in whom it presents as a painless testicular mass. Because benign testicular tumors are virtually nonexistent, biopsy is not done, and a radical orchiectomy is performed by the inguinal route. Blood samples are taken pre-op for serum markers (α-fetoprotein [AFP] and β-human chorionic gonadotropin [β-HCG]), which will be useful for follow-up. Further surgery for lymph node dissection may be done in some cases. Most testicular cancers are exquisitely radiosensitive and chemosensitive (platinum-based chemotherapy), offering many options for successful treatment in advanced, metastatic disease.

RETENTION AND INCONTINENCE

Acute urinary retention is very common in men who already have significant symptoms from benign prostatic hypertrophy. It is often precipitated during a cold, by the use of antihistamines and nasal drops, and abundant fluid intake. The patient wants to void but cannot, and the huge distended bladder is palpable.

- An indwelling bladder catheter needs to be placed and left in for at least 3 days.
- First line of long-term therapy is alpha-blockers. 5-alpha-reductase inhibitors are used for very large glands (>40 g).
- Minimally invasive procedures are under evaluation.
- The traditional transurethral resection of the prostate (TURP) is rarely done.

Postoperative urinary retention is also very common, and sometimes it masquerades as incontinence. The patient may not feel the need to void because of post-op pain, medications, etc., but will report that every few minutes there is involuntary release of small amounts of urine. A huge distended bladder will be palpable, confirming that the problem is overflow incontinence from retention. Indwelling bladder catheter is needed.

Stress incontinence is also very common in middle-aged women who have had many pregnancies and vaginal deliveries. They leak small amounts of urine whenever intra-abdominal pressure suddenly increases. This includes sneezing, laughing, getting out of a chair, or lifting a heavy object. They do not have any incontinence during the night. Examination will show a weak pelvic floor, with the prolapsed bladder neck outside of the "high-pressure" abdominal area.

- For early cases, pelvic floor exercises may be sufficient.
- For advanced cases with large cystoceles, surgical repair of the pelvic floor is indicated.
- For extreme cases, surgical reconstruction of the pelvic floor may be needed.

STONES

Passage of ureteral stones produces the classic colicky flank pain, with irradiation to the inner thigh and labia or scrotum, and sometimes nausea and vomiting. Most stones are visible on non-contrast CT scan. Although there is an array of fancy gadgetry available to deal with urinary stones, intervention is not always needed.

- Small stones (≤3 mm) at the ureterovesical junction have a 70% chance of passing spontaneously. Such cases can be handled with analgesics, plenty of fluids, and watchful waiting.
- On the other hand, a 7-mm stone at the UPJ only has a 5% probability of passing. Intervention will be required.

The most common tool used is extracorporeal shock-wave lithotripsy (ESWL). Sometimes ESWL cannot be used (pregnant women, bleeding diathesis, stones that are several centimeters large). Other options include basket extraction, sonic probes, laser beams, and open surgery. Although there is specific therapy for the prevention of recurrences in defined types of stones, abundant water intake is universally applicable.

MISCELLANEOUS

Pneumaturia is almost always caused by fistulization between the bladder and the GI tract, most commonly the sigmoid colon, and most commonly from diverticulitis (second possibility is cancer of the sigmoid, and cancer of the bladder is a very distant third). Workup starts with CT scan, which will show the inflammatory diverticular mass. Sigmoidoscopy is needed later to rule out cancer. Surgical therapy is required.

Impotence can be organic or psychogenic.

- **Psychogenic impotence** has sudden onset, is partner- or situation-specific, does not interfere with nocturnal erections (which can be tested with a roll of postage stamps), and can be effectively treated with psychotherapy only if it is done promptly.
- **Organic impotence**, if caused by trauma, will also have sudden onset, specifically related to the traumatic event (after pelvic surgery, because of nerve damage, or after trauma to the perineum, which involves arterial disruption).
  - Because of chronic disease (arteriosclerosis, diabetes), organic impotence has very gradual onset, going from erections not lasting long enough, to being of poor quality, to not happening at all (including absence of nocturnal erections).
  - Sildenafil, tadalafil, and vardenafil have become first choice therapy in many cases, but there are many other options, including vascular surgery (well-suited for those with arterial injury), suction devices (can be used on almost everybody), and prosthetic implants.

Organ Transplantation 13

Learning Objectives

❑ Describe the policies related to waiting lists for organ transplantation

❑ Describe the common complications in organ transplantation

Selection of donors has been liberalized tremendously to help alleviate the acute shortage of organs. Virtually all brain-dead patients are potential candidates, regardless of age. Donors with specific infections (e.g., hepatitis) can be used for recipients who have the same disease. Even donors with metastatic cancer can donate corneas.

The general rule for regular physicians is that all potential donors are referred to the harvesting teams, and they will exclude the few that cannot be used at all.

A positive HIV status is the only absolute contraindication to organ donation, though recent reports of donating to HIV+ recipients may change that policy.

Transplant rejection can happen in 3 ways: **hyperacute**, **acute**, and **chronic rejection**.

Hyperacute rejection is a vascular thrombosis that occurs within minutes of reestablishing blood supply to the organ. It is caused by preformed antibodies. It is prevented by ABO matching and lymphocytotoxic crossmatch, and thus it is not seen clinically.

Acute rejection (most common) occurs after the first 5 days, and usually within the first 3 months. Episodes occur even though the patient is on maintenance immunosuppression. Signs of organ dysfunction suggest it, and biopsy confirms it.

- In the case of the **liver**, technical problems are more commonly encountered than immunologic rejection. Thus, the first goal when liver function deteriorates post-transplant (rising g-glutamyltransferase [GGT], alkaline phosphatase, and bilirubin) is to rule out biliary obstruction by U/S and vascular thrombosis by Doppler.

- In the case of the **heart**, signs of functional deterioration occur too late to allow effective therapy, thus routine ventricular biopsies (by way of the jugular, superior vena cava, and right atrium) are done at set intervals. The first line of therapy for acute rejection is steroid boluses. If unsuccessful, antilymphocyte agents (OKT3) have been used though their high toxicity is a problem. Newer anti-thymocyte serum is tolerated better.

- Efforts are underway to come up with cellular MRI as a non-invasive way to diagnose rejection, without the need for biopsy. The field of allotransplantation is in continuous flux.

Chronic rejection is seen years after the transplant, with gradual, insidious loss of organ function. It is poorly understood and irreversible. Although we have no treatment for it, patients suspected of having it have the transplant biopsied in the hope that it may be a delayed (and treatable) case of acute rejection.

PART II

Surgical Vignettes

Trauma 1

PRIMARY SURVEY: THE ABCs

Airway

1. A patient involved in a car accident is fully conscious, and his voice is normal.

A very brief vignette, but in terms of the airway, the airway is fine.

2. A patient with multiple stab wounds arrives in the ED fully conscious, and he has a normal voice, but he also has an expanding hematoma in the neck.

3. A patient with multiple stab wounds arrives in the ED fully conscious, and he has a normal voice, but he also has subcutaneous air (emphysema) in the tissues in the neck and upper chest.

The airway may be fine now, but it is going to be compromised soon. Intubation is indicated now before an emergency situation develops. Orotracheal intubation with rapid-sequence anesthetic induction and pulse oximetry (or topical anesthesia) is preferred in the setting of a trauma center. Blind nasotracheal intubation is often performed by paramedics in the field. The patient with subcutaneous emphysema requires fiberoptic bronchoscopy (more details follow).

4. A patient involved in a severe car accident has multiple injuries and is unconscious. He is breathing spontaneously but his breathing sounds gurgled and noisy.

Altered mental status is the most common indication for intubation in the trauma patient. Unconscious patients with Glasgow coma scale ≤8 may not be able to maintain or protect their airway. Orotracheal intubation would be preferred here, but no anesthetic is needed.

5. An unconscious patient is brought in by the paramedics with spontaneous but noisy and labored breathing. They relate that at the accident site the patient was conscious, but was complaining of neck pain and was unable to move his lower extremities. He lost consciousness during the ambulance ride, and efforts to secure a nasotracheal airway were unsuccessful.

Although it is obvious that the patient has a cervical spine injury, his airway has to be managed first. Orotracheal intubation can still be performed with manual in-line cervical immobilization or over a flexible bronchoscope. Some prefer nasotracheal intubation in this setting if facial injuries do not preclude it.

6. A patient involved in a severe automobile crash is fully awake and alert, but he has extensive facial fractures and is bleeding briskly into his airway, and his voice is masked by gurgling sounds.

Securing an airway is mandatory, but the orotracheal route may not be suitable. Cricothyroidotomy is probably the best choice under these circumstances (except in the pediatric population because of the high-risk of airway stenosis in children, in whom a tracheostomy should be performed because the cricoid cartilage is much smaller than in the adult).

Breathing

7. An unconscious trauma patient has been rapidly intubated in the ER. He has spontaneous breathing and bilateral breath sounds, and his oxygen saturation by pulse oximetry is above 95.

As far as breathing is concerned, he is moving air (physical examination) and getting oxygen into his blood (oximetry). Deterioration could occur later, but right now we are ready to move to C in the ABCs.

Circulation

8. A 22-year-old man arrives in the ED with multiple gunshot wounds to the abdomen. He is diaphoretic, pale, cold, shivering, and anxious. He asks for a blanket and a drink of water. His BP is 60/40 mm Hg, pulse 150/min, and thready.

We recognize the picture of shock. In the trauma setting, shock is most commonly hypovolemic caused by bleeding, but other possibilities are pericardial tamponade or tension pneumothorax. Although each of these could occur with transabdominal gunshot wounds, it is less likely (than a direct thoracic injury), so most likely the source of shock is bleeding.

Management includes several simultaneous interventions:

- Large-bore IV lines
- Foley catheter
- Preparation of blood products for immediate exploratory laparotomy for control of bleeding
- Fluid and blood administration

The old emphasis on fluid resuscitation first has given way to a preference for control of the bleeding site as the first order of business, particularly when surgery will have to be done anyway. When surgery might or might not be needed as with blunt trauma, fluid resuscitation is still performed first, in part as a diagnostic test (patients who respond promptly and remain stable are probably no longer bleeding).

> 9. During a bank robbery an innocent bystander is shot multiple times in the abdomen. When the emergency medical technicians arrive, they find him to be in shock. A fully staffed trauma center is 2 miles away from the site of the shooting.

An ambulance can travel 2 miles in 2 minutes—maybe 3. The point of the vignette is that elaborate attempts to start an IV at the site and begin to infuse Ringer's lactate would waste precious time that would be best spent moving the patient to a place where the urgently needed laparotomy can be done ("scoop and run").

> 10. A 19-year-old male is shot in the right groin during a drug deal gone bad. He staggers to the hospital on his own, and arrives in the ED with BP 90/70 mm Hg and pulse 105/min. Bright red blood is squirting from the groin wound.

The point of this vignette is that control of the bleeding by direct local pressure is the first order of business before volume resuscitation is started. Finger pressure is used in the civilian setting, where typically there is a single patient and multiple health care workers. In the military combat setting, where the ratio is reversed, tourniquets are life-saving.

> 11. A car accident victim arrives at the ED both unconscious and with spontaneous but noisy breathing. His BP is 80/60 mm Hg, pulse 95/min. Head and neck veins are not obviously distended. While the anesthesia team is intubating him, another team is placing a central line for central venous pressure (CVP) measurement, and others are examining his chest and abdomen.

The emphasis on control of bleeding first and fluid replacement later cannot be implemented if we do not know yet where the bleeding is coming from, and whether it might stop spontaneously or not. In a case like this, two large (16-gauge) peripheral lines should be started, and Ringer's lactate should be rapidly infused.

At one time central venous lines were deemed essential for fluid resuscitation, but short, wide catheters in peripheral veins work better, and placing them does not interfere with other ongoing therapeutic and diagnostic maneuvers. Central lines should only be used when no other access is available or there is a need for monitoring. Percutaneous femoral vein catheter is an acceptable alternative when peripheral IVs are hard to start. Saphenous vein cut-downs, which were very popular in the 1950s, have also made a comeback as a suitable route.

12. A 4-year-old child has been shot in the arm in a drive-by shooting. The site of bleeding has been controlled by local pressure, but he is hypotensive and tachycardic. Two attempts at starting peripheral IVs have been unsuccessful.

Up to age 6, the access of last resort is intraosseous cannulation in the proximal tibia and femur. The initial bolus of Ringer's lactate would be 20 ml/kg of body weight.

13. During a wilderness trek, a 22-year-old man is attacked by a bear and bitten repeatedly in the arms and legs. His trek companion manages to kill the bear and to stop the bleeding by applying direct pressure, but when paramedics arrive 1 hour later, they find the patient to be in a state of shock. Transportation to the nearest hospital will take at least 2 hours.

All the training that paramedics took to enable them to infuse IV fluids has not been wasted. In the urban setting we now prefer rapid transportation to the hospital ("scoop and run"), but in this case prompt and vigorous fluid resuscitation is in order. The preferred fluid is Ringer's lactate, infusing at least 2 liters in the first 20–30 minutes.

14. A 22-year-old gang member arrives in the ED with multiple gunshot wounds to the chest and abdomen. He is diaphoretic, pale, cold, shivering, anxious, and asking for a blanket and a drink of water. His BP is 60/40 mm Hg and pulse 150/min and thready.

Hypovolemic shock is still the best bet, but the inclusion of chest wounds raises the possibility of pericardial tamponade or tension pneumothorax. As a rule, if significant findings are not included in the vignette, they are not present. Thus, as given, this is still a vignette of hypovolemic shock, but you may be offered in the answers the option of looking for the missing clinical signs: distended neck veins (or a high measured CVP) would be common to both tamponade and tension pneumothorax; and respiratory distress, tracheal deviation, and absent breath sounds on a hemithorax that is hyperresonant to percussion would specifically identify tension pneumothorax.

15. A 22-year-old gang member arrives in the ED with multiple gunshot wounds to the chest and abdomen. He is diaphoretic, pale, cold, shivering, anxious, and asking for a blanket and a drink of water. His BP is 60/40 mm Hg and pulse 150/min and thready. He has distended veins in his neck and forehead. He is breathing okay and has bilateral breath sounds and no tracheal deviation.

This is clearly describing the presentation of pericardial tamponade. Although the FAST exam or a formal transthoracic echocardiogram could confirm the diagnosis, it is clinically apparent and time is of the essence. Management entails evacuation of the blood in the pericardial space. This could be done by pericardiocentesis or pericardial window. If positive, follow with thoracotomy and then exploratory laparotomy. Fluid administration or blood transfusions would also help the patient with pericardial tamponade, but only as a temporizing measure while preparations are being made to evacuate the pericardial sac.

16. During a domestic dispute a young woman is stabbed in the chest with a 6-inch-long butcher knife. On arrival at the ED she is found to have an entry wound just to the left of the sternal border, at the fourth intercostal space. BP is 80/50 mm Hg and pulse 110/min. She is cold, pale, and perspiring heavily. She has big distended neck and facial veins, but she is breathing normally and has bilateral breath sounds.

There is no question that this is pericardial tamponade, and the location of the entry wound leaves no doubt as to the source: a stab wound to the heart. That will need to be repaired, and performing the median sternotomy will automatically open the pericardial sac and relieve the tamponade. Many trauma surgeons will not bother with previous pericardiocentesis or pericardial window, and will go straight to the OR.

17. A 22-year-old gang member arrives in the ED with multiple gunshot wounds to the chest and abdomen. He has labored breathing and is cyanotic, diaphoretic, cold, and shivering. His BP is 60/40 mm Hg and pulse 150/min and thready. He is in respiratory distress and has big distended veins in his neck and forehead, his trachea is deviated to the left, and the right side of his chest is hyperresonant to percussion, with no breath sounds.

This vignette describes a tension pneumothorax. Management entails immediate decompression using a large-bore needle or IV catheter placed into the right pleural space, followed by chest tube placement on the right side. Watch out for a trap which offers chest x-ray as an answer choice. Although this would confirm the diagnosis, it is clinically apparent and time is of the essence. Patient will die if sent to x-ray. Exploratory laparotomy will follow.

18. A 22-year-old man is involved in a high-speed, head-on automobile collision. He arrives in the ED in coma, with fixed, dilated pupils. He has multiple obvious fractures in both upper extremities and in the right lower leg. His BP is 70/50 mm Hg, with a barely perceptible pulse 140/min. His CVP is zero.

We have pointed out that shock in the trauma setting is caused by bleeding (the most common source), pericardial tamponade, or tension pneumothorax. This case fits right in, but the presence of obvious head injury might lead you into a trap: the question will offer you several kinds of intracranial bleeding (acute epidural hematoma, acute subdural hematoma, intracerebral bleeding, subarachnoid hemorrhage, etc.) as answer choices, all of which would be wrong. Intracranial bleeding can indeed kill you, but not by blood loss. There isn't enough room in the head to accommodate the amount of blood needed to go into shock (roughly a liter and a half in the average size adult). Thus, you need to look for another source (we will elaborate in the section on abdominal trauma).

19. A 72-year-old man who lives alone calls 911 saying that he has severe chest pain. He cannot give a coherent history when picked up by the EMTs, and on arrival at the ED he is cold and diaphoretic and his BP is 80/65mm Hg. He has an irregular, feeble pulse at 130/min. His neck and forehead veins are distended, and he is short of breath.

Many findings are similar to above cases but in the absence of trauma: old man, chest pain, straightforward cardiogenic shock from massive MI. Management entails electrocardiogram (ECG), check coronary enzymes, admit to coronary care unit, etc. Do not drown him with enthusiastic fluid "resuscitation," but use thrombolytic therapy if offered.

20. A 17-year-old girl is stung many times by a swarm of bees. On arrival to the ED she has BP 75/20 mm Hg and pulse 150/min, but she looks warm and flushed rather than pale and cold. CVP is low.

21. Twenty minutes after receiving a penicillin injection, a man breaks into hives and develops wheezing. On arrival at the ED his BP 75/20 mm Hg and pulse 150/min, but he looks warm and flushed rather than pale and cold. CVP is low.

22. In preparation for an inguinal hernia repair, a patient has a spinal anesthetic placed. His level of sensory block is much higher than anticipated, and shortly thereafter his BP becomes 75/20 mm Hg, but he looks warm and flushed rather than pale and cold. CVP is low.

All of these vignettes describe vasomotor shock due to anaphylaxis or inhibition of the sympathetic nervous system. Management is vasoconstrictors and volume replacement.

A REVIEW FROM HEAD TO TOE

Head Trauma

1. An 18-year-old man arrives in the ED with an ax firmly implanted into his head. Although it is clear from the size of the ax blade and the penetration that he has sustained an intracranial wound, he is awake and alert and hemodynamically stable.

The management of penetrating wounds is fairly straightforward. There will be exceptions, but as a rule the damage done to the internal organs (in this case the brain) will need to be repaired surgically. This man will go to the OR, and it will be there, under anesthesia and with full control, that the ax will be removed. An important detail when the weapon is embedded in the patient and part of it is sticking out is not to remove it in the ED or at the scene of the accident.

2. In the course of a mugging, a man is hit over the head with a blunt instrument. He has a scalp laceration, and CT scan shows an underlying linear skull fracture. He is neurologically intact and gives no history of having lost consciousness.

The rule in skull fractures is that if they are closed (no overlying wound) and asymptomatic, they are left alone. If they are open (like this one), the laceration has to be cleaned and closed, but if not comminuted or depressed, it can be done in the ER.

3. In the course of a mugging, a man is hit over the head with a blunt instrument. He has a scalp laceration, and CT scan shows an underlying comminuted, depressed skull fracture. He is neurologically intact and gives no history of having lost consciousness.

This one goes to the OR for cleaning and repair, and possible craniotomy.

4. A pedestrian is hit by a car. When brought to the ED he has minor bruises and lacerations but is otherwise quite well, with a completely normal neurologic exam. However, the ambulance crew reports that he was unconscious at the site, and although he woke up during the ambulance ride and is now completely lucid, he does not remember how the accident happened.

Anyone who has been hit over the head and has become unconscious gets a CT scan, looking for intracranial hematomas. If the CT scan and the neurologic exam are normal, he can go home—provided his family is willing to wake him up frequently over the next 24 hours to make sure he is not going into coma.

5. A pedestrian is hit by a car. He arrives in the ED in coma. He has ecchymosis around both eyes (raccoon eyes).

6. A pedestrian is hit by a car. He arrives in the ED in coma. He has clear fluid dripping out of his nose.

7. A pedestrian is hit by a car. He arrives in the ED in coma. He has clear fluid dripping from the ear.

8. A pedestrian is hit by a car. He arrives in the ED in coma. He has ecchymosis behind the ear.

Cases 5–8 are vignettes of basal skull fracture; they all require CT scan because the patient is in a coma. The scan will show the fractures, but nothing will actually be done about them. Typically, the leak of CSF will stop by itself, and although there is a higher risk of meningitis, prophylactic antibiotics have not proven to be of use. The CT scan should be extended to include the neck because the most important feature of these 4 vignettes is that the patients sustained significant trauma to the head and thus are at risk for lesions of the cervical spine.

9. A 14-year-old boy is hit over the side of the head with a baseball bat. He loses consciousness for a few minutes, but he recovers promptly and continues to play. One hour later he is found unconscious in the locker room. His right pupil is fixed and dilated. There are signs of contralateral hemiparesis.

This vignette describes an acute epidural hematoma, most likely on the right side. Diagnosis is made with CT scan, which will show a lens-shaped hematoma and deviation of the midline structures to the opposite side. Management is emergency surgical decompression via craniotomy. It has a good prognosis if treated, but fatal within hours if it is not.

10. A 32-year-old man is involved in a head-on, high-speed automobile collision. He is unconscious at the site, regains consciousness briefly during the ambulance ride, and arrives at the ED in deep coma with a fixed, dilated right pupil and contralateral hemiparesis.

This could be an acute epidural hematoma, but acute subdural is a better bet (big-time trauma, sicker patient). Diagnosis is made with CT scan, which will show a semilunar, crescent-shaped hematoma. Given the lateralizing signs, it will also show deviation of the midline structures to the opposite side. Be sure to check the cervical spine also!

Management requires an emergency craniotomy with evacuation of the clot often leading to significant improvement, particularly when the brain is being pushed to the side, but ultimate prognosis is poor because of accompanying parenchymal injury.

11. A man involved in a high-speed, head-on automobile collision is in coma. He has never had any lateralizing signs, and CT scan shows a small crescent shaped hematoma, but there is no deviation of the midline structures.

Another subdural hematoma, but without lateralizing signs and evidence of displacement of the midline structures, surgery has little to offer. Management will probably be directed at controlling ICP, as detailed in the next vignette.

12. A patient involved in a head-on, high-speed automobile collision arrives in the ED in deep coma, with bilateral fixed dilated pupils. CT scan of the head shows diffuse blurring of the gray-white mass interface and multiple small punctate hemorrhages. There is no single large hematoma or displacement of the midline structures.

The CT findings are classic for diffuse axonal injury. Prognosis is terrible, and surgery cannot help. Therapy will be directed at preventing further injury from increased ICP. Probably ICP monitoring will be in order. First-line measures to lower ICP include head elevation, hyperventilation, and avoidance of fluid overload. Mannitol and furosemide are next in line.

Do not overdo the treatment. Lowering ICP is not the ultimate goal; preserving brain perfusion is. Thus, diuretics which lead to systemic hypotension, or measures which produce excessive cerebral vasoconstriction may be counterproductive. Hyperventilation is indicated when there are clinical signs of herniation, and the goal is PCO_2 of 35. Lowering oxygen demand may also help. Sedation has been used for that purpose, and hypothermia is currently advocated for the same reason.

13. A 77-year-old man "becomes senile" over a period of 3 or 4 weeks. He used to be active and managed all of his financial affairs. Now he stares at the wall, barely talks, and sleeps most of the day. His daughter recalls that he fell from a horse about a week before the mental changes began.

This vignette is suspicious for a chronic subdural hematoma due to venous bleeding. Diagnosis is made with CT scan, and management is surgical decompression via craniotomy. Spectacular improvement is expected if recognized and treated appropriately.

14. A 45-year-old man is involved in a high-speed automobile collision. He arrives at the ED in coma with fixed, dilated pupils. He has multiple other injuries, including fractures of the extremities. His BP is 70/50 mm Hg with a feeble pulse 130/min. What kind of intracranial bleeding is responsible for the low BP and high pulse rate?

This very same vignette was presented in the review of shock. Shock does not result from intracranial bleeding (not enough room in the head for sufficient blood loss to cause shock). Look for an answer of significant blood loss to the outside (could be scalp laceration), or inside (abdomen, pelvic fractures).

Neck Trauma

15. A man has been shot in the neck and his BP is rapidly deteriorating.

Not much detail, but the point is that penetrating wounds anywhere in the neck need immediate surgical exploration if the patient is unstable (i.e., if vital signs are deteriorating).

16. A 42-year-old man is shot once with a .22-caliber revolver. The entrance wound is in the anterior left side of the neck, at the level of the thyroid cartilage. X-rays show that the bullet is embedded in the right scalene muscle. He is spitting and coughing blood and has an expanding hematoma under the entrance wound. His BP responded promptly to fluid administration, and he has remained stable.

A clear-cut case of a penetrating wound in the middle of the neck (zone II) that has alarming symptoms and therefore follows the rule (rather than the exception) for all penetrating injuries: immediate surgical exploration is required. This is true even though he is stable. The middle of the neck is packed with structures that should not have holes in them and are easily accessible via surgical exploration.

17. A young man is shot in the upper part of the neck. Evaluation of the entrance and exit wounds indicates that the trajectory is all above the level of the angle of the mandible. A steady trickle of blood flows from both wounds, and does not seem to respond to local pressure. The patient is drunk and combative but seems to be otherwise stable.

Now we are getting into the exceptions. In this very high level of the neck (Zone III) there is no trachea or esophagus to worry about, but only pharynx—injuries to which are less consequential. Vascular injuries are the only potential problem, but getting to them surgically is not easy. Thus angiography is a better choice, both for diagnosis and potentially for embolization.

18. A young man suffers a gunshot wound to the base of his neck. The entrance and exit wounds are above the clavicles but below the cricoid cartilage. He is hemodynamically stable.

This is another part of the neck (Zone I, or the thoracic outlet) that is crammed with vital structures that should be promptly repaired if they are injured. But precise preoperative diagnosis would help plan the incision and surgical approach. If the patient is stable, the standard workup includes angiography, soluble-contrast esophagogram, esophagoscopy, and bronchoscopy.

19. In the course of a bar fight, a young man is stabbed once in the neck. The entrance wound is in front of the sternomastoid muscle on the right, at the level of the thyroid cartilage. The patient is completely asymptomatic, and his vital signs are completely normal.

In stab wounds to the upper and middle zones of the neck, completely asymptomatic patients can be closely observed but investigate if any symptoms arise.

20. A patient who was the unbelted right front-seat passenger in a car flies through the windshield when the car crashes into a telephone pole at 30 miles an hour. He arrives in the ED strapped to a headboard and with sandbags on both sides of the neck. He has multiple facial lacerations but is otherwise stable.

    Examination of the neck reveals persistent pain and tenderness to palpation over the posterior midline of the neck. Neurologic examination is normal.

Every patient with head injuries from blunt trauma is at risk for cervical spine injury. The paramedics transport everyone as if they had such injury. Neurologic deficits provide a clear answer (more about those later), but in the patient who arrives neurologically intact, we don't want to make the diagnosis by allowing neurologic deficits to develop. Persistent local pain over the suspected area should trigger radiologic evaluation, which is best done with a CT scan of the neck.

Spinal Cord Injury

21. An 18-year-old street fighter gets stabbed in the back, just to the right side of the midline. He has paralysis and loss of proprioception distal to the injury on the right side, and loss of pain perception distal to the injury on the left side.

Probably no one in real life will have such a neat, clear-cut syndrome, but for purposes of the exam this is a classic spinal cord hemisection, better known as Brown-Séquard syndrome.

22. A patient involved in a car accident sustains a burst fracture of the vertebral bodies. He develops loss of motor function and loss of pain and temperature sensation on both sides distal to the injury, while showing preservation of vibratory sense and position.

Anterior cord syndrome.

23. An elderly man is involved in a rear-end automobile collision in which he hyperextends his neck. He develops paralysis and burning pain on both upper extremities while maintaining good motor function in his legs.

Central cord syndrome.

Management for cases 21–23 requires making the precise diagnosis. CT scans are good to look at the cervical bones. To evaluate the cord, MRI is better. Beyond that, the specific and complicated management of spinal cord injuries is unlikely to be tested on the examination.

Chest Trauma

24. A 75-year-old man slips and falls at home, hitting his right chest wall against the kitchen counter. He has an area of exquisite pain to direct palpation over the seventh rib, at the level of the anterior axillary line. Chest x-ray confirms the presence of a rib fracture, with no other abnormal findings.

A plain rib fracture is the most common chest injury. It is bothersome but manageable in most people, but it can be hazardous in the elderly as splinting and hypoventilation leads to atelectasis and can ultimately lead to pneumonia. The key to treatment is local pain relief, best achieved by nerve block and epidural catheter. Beware of the wrong answers that call for strapping or binding.

25. A 25-year-old man is stabbed in the right chest. He is moderately short of breath and has stable vital signs. There are no breath sounds on the right, which is hyperresonant to percussion.

This vignette describes an uncomplicated pneumothorax. Diagnosis is made with chest x-ray; is this case, as opposed to a tension pneumothorax, there is time to get an x-ray if the option is offered. Ultimately, management is with insertion of a chest tube. If given an option for location, it should be placed at the fifth intercostal space in the mid-axillary line, above the rib.

26. A 25-year-old man is stabbed in the right chest. He is moderately short of breath and has stable vital signs. The base of the right chest has no breath sounds and is dull to percussion. He has faint distant breath sounds at the apex.

Given these findings, this case sounds more like hemothorax. Diagnosis is again made with chest x-ray, and if confirmed, treatment is still with a chest tube. This allows drainage to enable ventilation, assess quantity of bleeding, and drain blood because if blood is allowed to remain in the pleural space, it will lead to adhesions and form a fibrothorax or get infected and create an empyema.

27. A 25-year-old man is stabbed in the right chest. He is moderately short of breath and has stable vital signs. There are no breath sounds at the right base, and only faint distant breath sounds at the apex. The right base is dull to percussion. Chest x-ray confirms the presence of a hemothorax. A chest tube placed at the right pleural base recovers 120 ml of blood and drains another 20 ml in the next hour.

The point of this case is that most hemothoraces do not need exploratory surgery. Bleeding is typically from the lung parenchyma (low pressure) and stops by itself. It also can be from the intercostal artery. A chest tube is all that is needed. Key clue: little blood retrieved, even less afterward.

28. A 25-year-old man is stabbed in the right chest. He is moderately short of breath, has BP of 95/70 mm Hg, pulse 100/min. No breath sounds are heard over the right chest, which is dull to percussion. Chest x-ray shows a large hemothorax on the right. A chest tube placed at the right pleural base recovers 1,250 ml of blood.

The exception is bleeding from a systemic vessel or a major vessel in the pulmonary circuit which will need surgical exploration to repair or ligate. The most likely culprit is an intercostal artery. One or more of the following is required for proceeding with surgical exploration:

- Immediate drainage >1.5 L
- >250 mL/hour for 4 hours
- Hemodynamic instability with high output

29. A 25-year-old man is stabbed in the right chest. He is moderately short of breath and has stable vital signs. There are no breath sounds at the right base, and only faint distant breath sounds at the apex. The right base is dull to percussion. Chest x-ray confirms the presence of a hemothorax. A chest tube placed at the right pleural base recovers 350 ml of blood. Over the ensuing 4 hours he continues to drain 200–300 mL of blood/hour.

Another example of bleeding from a systemic vessel (most likely an intercostal) that will require a thoracotomy.

30. A 25-year-old man is stabbed in the right chest. He is moderately short of breath, has stable vital signs. No breath sounds on the right. Hyperresonant to percussion at the apex of the right chest, dull at the base. Chest x-ray shows one single, large air-fluid level.

This describes a hemopneumothorax. Chest tube placement would ideally be at the base to make sure all the blood is drained. Subsequent management criteria as in the previous vignettes.

31. A worker has been injured at an explosion in a factory. He has multiple cuts and lacerations from flying debris, and he is obviously short of breath. The paramedics at the scene of the accident ascertain that he has a large, flaplike wound in the chest wall, about 5 cm in diameter, and he sucks air through it with every inspiratory effort.

The classic sucking chest wound. It needs to be covered to prevent further air intake (Vaseline gauze is ideal), but must be allowed to let air out. Taping the dressing on 3 sides creates a one-way flap that allows air to escape but not enter. Once in the hospital, he will need a chest tube.

32. A 54-year-old woman crashes her car against a telephone pole at high speed. On arrival at the ED she is in moderate respiratory distress. She has multiple bruises on the chest, and multiple sites of point tenderness over the ribs. X-rays show multiple rib fractures on both sides. On closer observation it is noted that a segment of chest wall on the left side caves in when she inhales, and bulges out when she exhales.

Paradoxical breathing as described essentially makes the diagnosis of flail chest. Diagnosis is easy, but management requires a long discussion. Management of severe blunt trauma to the chest from a deceleration injury has 3 components:

- Treatment of the obvious lesion
- Monitoring for other pathology that may not become obvious until a day or two later
- Actively investigating the potential presence of a silent killer, traumatic transection of the aorta

In this case, the obvious lesion is flail chest. The problem there is the underlying pulmonary contusion, which is treated with fluid restriction, diuretics, and close monitoring of blood gases. Should blood gases deteriorate, the patient needs to be placed on a respirator and get bilateral chest tubes (because lungs punctured by the broken ribs could leak air once positive pressure ventilation is started, which could lead to a tension pneumothorax).

Monitoring is needed over the next 48 hours for possible signs of pulmonary or myocardial contusion. Repeated chest x-rays, blood gases, EKGs, and troponins are needed.

Traumatic transection of the aorta is best diagnosed with CTA of the chest.

33. A 54-year-old woman crashes her car into a telephone pole at high speed. On arrival at the ED she is breathing well. She has multiple bruises over the chest, and multiple sites of point tenderness over the ribs. X-rays show multiple rib fractures on both sides, but the lung parenchyma is clear and both lungs are expanded. Two days later her lungs "white out" on x-rays and she is in respiratory distress.

This is a classic presentation of pulmonary contusion. It does not always show up right away, may become evident 1 or 2 days after the trauma. Management consists of fluid restriction, diuretics, and respiratory support. The latter is essential with intubation, mechanical ventilation, and PEEP if needed.

34. A 33-year-old woman is involved in a high-speed automobile collision. She arrives at the ED gasping for breath, cyanotic at the lips, with flaring nostrils. There are bruises over both sides of the chest, and tenderness suggestive of multiple fractured ribs. BP is 60/45 mm Hg and pulse 160/min and thready. She has distended neck and forehead veins and is diaphoretic. Her left hemithorax has no breath sounds and is hyperresonant to percussion.

A variation on an old theme: classic picture for tension pneumothorax—but where is the penetrating trauma? The fractured ribs can act as a penetrating weapon.

Management. Needle through the upper anterior chest wall to decompress the pleural space, followed by chest tube on the left. Do not fall for the option of getting x-ray first, though you need it later to verify the correct position of the chest tube. This is a deceleration injury. You also need to look for traumatic transection of the aorta with a CTA as discussed.

35. A 54-year-old woman crashes her car against a telephone pole at high speed. On arrival at the ED she is breathing well. She has multiple bruises over the chest, and is exquisitely tender over the sternum at a point where there is a gritty feeling of bone grating on bone, elicited by palpation.

Obviously this describes a sternal fracture (which a lateral chest x-ray will confirm), but the point is that she is at high risk for myocardial contusion and for traumatic rupture of the aorta. Diagnosis of cardiac contusion is made by ECG, and management of arrhythmias as they develop. Serum troponin levels are not always useful as they will not change management. But the real important test would be CTA looking for an aortic rupture given the mechanism of injury.

36. A 53-year-old man is involved in a high-speed automobile collision. He has moderate respiratory distress. Physical examination shows no breath sounds over the entire left chest. Percussion is unremarkable. Chest x-ray shows multiple air fluid levels in the left chest.

This is classic for traumatic diaphragmatic rupture with resultant migration of intra-abdominal contents into the left chest; the right side is protected by the liver so it always occurs to the left.

A nasogastric (NG) tube curling up into the left chest might be an added tidbit. In suspicious cases, laparoscopic evaluation is indicated. Management is surgical repair either through the abdomen (more common) or chest dependent on the surgeon

37. A motorcycle daredevil attempts to jump over the 12 fountains in front of Caesar's Palace Hotel in Las Vegas. As he leaves the ramp at very high speed, his motorcycle turns sideways and he hits the retaining wall at the other end, literally like a rag doll. At the ED he is found to be remarkably stable, although he has multiple extremity fractures. Chest x-ray shows fracture of the left first rib and widened mediastinum.

What is it? This is a real case. Classic for traumatic rupture of the aorta: massive trauma, fracture of a hard-to-break bone (could be first rib, scapula, or sternum), and the telltale hint of widened mediastinum.

Diagnosis is with spiral CT scan. Management is emergency surgical repair.

38. A 34-year-old woman suffers severe blunt trauma in a car accident. She has multiple injuries to her extremities, head trauma, and pneumothorax on the left side. Shortly after initial examination it is noted that she is developing progressive subcutaneous emphysema all over her upper chest and lower neck.

Three things can give thoracic subcutaneous emphysema. One is rupture of the esophagus, but the setting there is always after endoscopy (for which it is diagnostic). The second one is tension pneumothorax, but there the alarming findings are all the others already reviewed—the emphysema is barely a footnote. That leaves the third (which is the case): traumatic rupture of the trachea or major bronchus.

Diagnosis is with chest x-ray to confirm the presence of air in the tissues. Fiberoptic bronchoscopy will confirm diagnosis and level of injury and to secure an airway. Surgical repair thereafter.

39. A patient who had received a chest tube for a traumatic pneumothorax is noted to be putting out a very large amount of air through the tube (a large air leak), and his collapsed lung is not expanding.

Another presentation for a major bronchial injury.

40. A patient who sustained a penetrating injury of the chest has been intubated and placed on a respirator, and a chest tube has been placed in the appropriate pleural cavity. The patient had been hemodynamically stable throughout, but then suddenly goes into cardiac arrest.

A typical scenario for air embolism, from an injured bronchus to a nearby injured pulmonary vein, and from there to the left ventricle. Immediate management includes cardiac massage, followed by thoracotomy.

41. During the performance of a supraclavicular node biopsy under local anesthesia, suddenly a hissing sound is heard, and the patient drops dead.

42. A patient who is receiving total parenteral nutrition through a central venous line becomes frustrated because the nurses are not answering his call button, so he gets up and out of bed, and disconnects his central line from the IV tubing. With the open catheter dangling, he takes two steps in the direction of the nurses station, and drops dead.

Two more examples of air embolism. Other thoracic calamities such as tension pneumothorax or continued bleeding will produce severe deterioration of vital signs, but there will be a sequence from being okay to becoming terribly ill. When vignettes give you sudden death, think of air embolism. This is very uncommon.

43. A patient who sustained severe blunt trauma, including multiple fractures of long bones, becomes disoriented about 12 hours after admission. Shortly thereafter he develops petechial rashes in the axillae and neck, fever, and tachycardia. A few hours later he has a full-blown picture of respiratory distress with hypoxemia. Chest x-ray shows bilateral patchy infiltrates, and his platelet count is low.

This is not a chest injury, but is included here because its main problem is respiratory distress. You probably recognized already the fat embolism syndrome. It is not clear how specific the lab finding of fat droplets in the urine is, but it does not matter: the mainstay of therapy is respiratory support—which is needed regardless of the etiology of the respiratory distress. Heparin, steroids, alcohol, and low-molecular-weight dextran have all been used, but are of questionable value.

Abdominal Trauma

44. A 19-year-old gang member is shot in the abdomen with a .38-caliber revolver. The entry wound is in the epigastrium, to the left of the midline. The bullet is lodged in the psoas muscle on the right. He is hemodynamically stable, the abdomen is moderately tender.

No diagnostic tests are needed. A penetrating gunshot wound of the abdomen gets exploratory laparotomy every time. Preparations before surgery include an indwelling bladder catheter, a large-bore venous line for fluid administration, and a dose of broad-spectrum antibiotics.

45. At exploratory laparotomy for the patient described in the previous question, examination shows clean, punched-out entrance and exit wounds in the transverse colon.

If there is gross fecal contamination, do a colostomy. With minimal contamination, primary repair is usually okay.

46. A 19-year-old gang member is shot once with a .38-caliber revolver. The entry wound is in the left mid-clavicular line, 2 inches below the nipple. The bullet is lodged in the left paraspinal muscles. He is hemodynamically stable, but he is drunk and combative and physical examination is difficult to perform.

What is it? The point here is to remind you of the boundaries of the abdomen; though this seems like a chest wound, it is also abdominal. The belly begins at the nipple line. The chest does not end at the nipple line, though. Belly and chest are not stacked up like pancakes: they are separated by a dome. This patient needs all the stuff for a penetrating chest wound (chest x-ray, chest tube if needed), plus the exploratory laparotomy.

47. A 42-year-old man is stabbed in the belly by a jealous lover. The wound is lateral to the umbilicus, on the left, and omentum can be seen protruding through it.

The general rule is that penetrating abdominal wounds get a laparotomy. That is true for gunshot wounds, but it is also true for stab wounds if it is clear that peritoneal penetration took place.

48. In the course of a domestic fight, a 38-year-old obese woman is attacked with a 4-inch-long switchblade. In addition to several superficial lacerations, she was stabbed in the abdomen. She is hemodynamically stable, and does not have any signs of peritoneal irritation.

This is probably the only exception to the rule that penetrating abdominal wounds have to be surgically explored—and that is because this in fact may not be penetrating at all! (The blade was short, the woman is well padded.) Local wound exploration of the wound tract in the ED may show that no abdominal surgery is needed (i.e. the anterior rectus fascia has not been violated). But if there is any suspicion of intra-abdominal injury, obtain an abdominal CT.

49. A 31-year-old woman smashes her car against a wall. She has multiple injuries including upper and lower extremity fractures. Her BP is 75/55 mm Hg, pulse rate 110/min, and CVP 0. On physical examination she has a tender abdomen, with guarding and rebound on all quadrants.

50. A 31-year-old woman smashes her car against a wall. She has multiple injuries including upper and lower extremity fractures. Her BP is 135/75 mm Hg and pulse 82/min. On physical examination she has a tender abdomen, with guarding and rebound on all quadrants.

Solid organs will bleed when smashed. Hollow viscera will spill their contents. Often they both happen, but one can exist without the other. Here we have 2 vignettes with plenty of clues to suggest that abnormal fluid is loose in the belly. In one case there is also bleeding, in the other there is not; but the presence of "acute abdomen" after blunt abdominal trauma mandates laparotomy. They will both need it.

51. A 26-year-old woman has been involved in a car wreck. She has fractures in both upper extremities, facial lacerations, and no other obvious injuries. Chest x-ray is normal. Shortly thereafter she develops hypotension, tachycardia, and dropping hematocrit. Her CVP is low.

Obviously blood loss, but the question is where. The answer is easy: it has to be in the abdomen. To go into hypovolemic shock one has to lose 25–30% of blood volume, which in the average size adult will be nearly 1.5 L (25–30% of 5 L).

In the absence of external hemorrhage (scalp lacerations can bleed that much), the bleeding has to be internal. That much blood cannot fit inside the head, and would not go unnoticed in the neck (huge hematoma) or chest (a good decubitus x-ray can spot anything >150 ml, and even in other positions 1.5 L would be obvious). Only massive pelvic fractures, multiple femur fractures, or intra-abdominal bleeding can accommodate that much blood. The first two would be evident in physical examination and x-rays. The belly can be silent. Thus the belly is invariably the place to look for that hidden blood.

Diagnosis. We have a choice here. The old, invasive way was the diagnostic peritoneal lavage. The newer, noninvasive ways are the CT scan or sonogram. CT scan is best, but it cannot be done in the patient who is "crashing." (The exam questions still assume that fast CT scanners are not available in every emergency department in the nation. Under this assumption, only hemodynamically stable patients can get the CT scan.) Try to gauge from the question whether the patient is stable—do CT scan—or literally dying on your hands, in which case diagnostic peritoneal lavage or sonogram is performed in the ED or the OR.

Management. Most likely finding will be ruptured spleen. If stable, observation with serial hemoglobin and hematocrit levels every 6 hours for 48 hours. If not, exploratory laparotomy.

52. A 27-year-old intoxicated man smashes his car against a tree. He is tender over the left lower chest wall. Chest x-ray shows fractures of the 8th, 9th, and 10th ribs on the left. He has a BP of 85 over 68 and a pulse rate 128/min, which do not respond satisfactorily to fluid and blood administration. He has a positive peritoneal lavage, and at exploratory laparotomy a ruptured spleen is found.

You are unlikely to be asked technical surgical questions, but when dealing with a ruptured spleen, remove it. Further management includes administration of Pneumovax and also immunization for *Haemophilus influenza* B and meningococcus.

53. A multiple trauma patient is receiving massive blood transfusions as the surgeons are attempting to repair many intraabdominal injuries. It is then noted that blood is oozing from all dissected raw surfaces, as well as from his IV line sites. His core temperature is normal.

Signs of coagulopathy in this setting require a shotgun approach to treatment. Empiric administration of both fresh-frozen plasma and platelet packs is recommended, in a 1:1 ratio with packed RBCs.

54. During the course of a laparotomy for multiple trauma, the patient develops a significant coagulopathy, a core temperature below 34°C, and refractory acidosis.

This combination of hypothermia, coagulopathy, and acidosis is referred to as the "triad of death." It requires that the abdomen be packed and temporarily closed immediately (as long as major vascular injuries and GI tract injuries leading to contamination have been controlled).

55. An exploratory laparotomy for multiple intraabdominal injuries has lasted 3.5 hours, during which time multiple blood transfusions have been given, and several liters of Ringer's lactate have been infused. When the surgeons are ready to close the abdomen they find that the abdominal wall edges cannot be pulled together without undue tension. Both the belly wall and the abdominal contents seem to be swollen.

This is the abdominal compartment syndrome. All the fluid that has been infused has kept the patient alive, but at the expense of creating a lot of edema in the operative area. Forced closure would produce all kinds of problems. The bowel cannot be left exposed to the outside either, so the standard approach is to close the wound with an absorbable mesh over which formal closure can be done later, or with a nonabsorbable plastic cover that will be removed later.

56. In postoperative day 1, a trauma patient develops a very tense and distended abdomen, and the retention sutures are cutting through the abdominal wall. He also develops hypoxia and renal failure.

This is also the abdominal compartment syndrome that was not obvious at the end of the operation, but has developed thereafter. The abdomen will have to be decompressed by opening the incision and using a temporary cover as described above.

Pelvic Fracture

57. In a rollover motor vehicle accident, a 42-year-old woman is thrown out of the car and subsequently becomes crushed underneath it. At evaluation in the ED it is determined that she has a pelvic fracture. She arrived hypotensive, but responded promptly to fluid administration. CT scan shows no intraabdominal bleeding but a pelvic hematoma.

Nonexpanding pelvic hematomas in a patient who has become hemodynamically stable are left alone. Depending on the type of fracture, the orthopedic surgeons may eventually do something to stabilize the pelvis, but at this time the main issue is to rule out the potential associated pelvic injuries: rectum, bladder, and vagina. Physical examination and a Foley catheter will do it.

58. In a rollover motor vehicle accident, a 42-year-old woman is thrown out of the car and subsequently becomes crushed underneath it. At evaluation in the ED it is determined that she has a pelvic fracture. She arrived hypotensive but did not respond to fluid resuscitation. Hemodynamic parameters have continued to deteriorate. FAST exam performed at the ED shows no intraabdominal bleeding.

A tough situation. People can bleed to death from pelvic fracture so it makes sense to do something about it. But that is easier said than done. Surgical exploration is not the answer; these injuries are typically not in the surgical field afforded by a laparotomy. Ateriographic evaluation might reveal arterial bleeding amenable to embolization. Angiographic therapy is not effective for venous bleeding. External pelvic fixation might be the only helpful intervention. A reasonable sequence to give in the examination, as the answer to this vignette, would be external pelvic fixation first, followed by a trip to the angiography suite (interventional radiology) for possible angiographic embolization of both internal iliac arteries.

Urologic Injury

59. A young man is shot point blank in the lower abdomen, just above the pubis. He has blood in the urine, and no evidence of rectal injury.

60. A woman is shot in the flank, and when a Foley catheter was inserted in ED, the urine was found to be grossly bloody.

The hallmark of urologic injuries is blood in the urine after trauma. These two are clear-cut. The therapy is also clear. Penetrating urologic injuries are like most penetrating injuries elsewhere: they need surgical repair.

61. A 22-year-old man involved in a high-speed automobile collision has multiple injuries, including a pelvic fracture. On physical examination there is blood at the meatus.

What is it? The vignette will be longer, but the point is that pelvic fracture plus blood at the meatus in a male means either bladder or urethral injury, most likely the latter. Evaluation starts with a retrograde urethrogram because urethral injury would be compounded by insertion of a Foley catheter.

62. A 19-year-old man is involved in a severe automobile accident. Among many other injuries he has a pelvic fracture. He has blood at the meatus, scrotal hematoma, and the sensation that he wants to urinate but cannot. Rectal examination shows a high-riding prostate.

What is it? This is a more complete description of a posterior urethral injury.

Diagnosis. You already know: retrograde urethrogram.

63. A 19-year-old man is involved in a motorcycle accident. Among many other injuries he has a pelvic fracture. He has blood at the meatus and scrotal hematoma.

This is an anterior urethral injury.

64. A 22-year-old man involved in a high-speed automobile collision has multiple injuries, including a pelvic fracture. At the initial physical examination no blood is seen at the meatus. A poorly informed intern attempts insertion of a Foley catheter, but resistance is met.

Back out! Although the blood at the meatus or the perineal hematoma were not there to warn you, this is also a urethral injury. Do the retrograde urethrogram.

65. A 22-year-old woman involved in a high-speed automobile collision has multiple injuries, including a pelvic fracture. Insertion of a Foley catheter reveals gross hematuria.

What is it? It most likely is a bladder injury.

Assessment will require retrograde cystogram or CT cystography. When done, obvious intraperitoneal extravasation may be seen (rupture at the dome), but if "negative" you need another film after the bladder is empty. Ruptures at the trigone leak retroperitoneally, and the leak may be obscured by the bladder full of dye.

66. A patient involved in a high-speed automobile collision has multiple injuries, including rib fractures and abdominal contusions (but no pelvic fracture). Insertion of a Foley catheter shows that there is gross hematuria.

What is it? The blood most likely is coming from the kidneys.

Diagnosis is with CT scan. For management, the rule is that traumatic hematuria from blunt trauma to the kidney does not need surgery, even if the kidney is smashed. Surgery is done only if the renal pedicle is avulsed or the patient is exsanguinating.

67. A patient involved in a high-speed automobile collision has multiple injuries, including rib fractures and abdominal contusions. Insertion of a Foley catheter shows that there is hematuria, and retrograde cystogram is normal. CT scan shows renal injuries that do not require surgery. Six weeks later the patient develops acute shortness of breath and a flank bruit.

What is it? This is a weird one, but so fascinating that some medical school professors may not be able to resist the temptation to include it. The patient developed a traumatic arteriovenous fistula at the renal pedicle, and subsequent heart failure. Management is arteriogram and surgical correction.

68. A 35-year-old man is about to be discharged from the hospital where he was under observation for multiple blunt trauma sustained in a car wreck. It is then discovered that he has microscopic hematuria.

69. A 4-year-old falls off his tricycle. In the ensuing evaluation he is found to have microscopic hematuria.

Gross traumatic hematuria always has to be investigated, in both children and adults, while microscopic hematuria following trauma does not. At one time it was felt that microscopic hematuria following trauma in children was suggestive of congenital abnormalities and thus deserved mandatory investigation. That is no longer considered absolute. Obviously, any kind of hematuria—needs to be followed.

70. A 14-year-old boy slides down a banister, not realizing that there is a big knob at the end of it. He smashes the scrotum and comes to the ED with a scrotal hematoma the size of a grapefruit. He can urinate normally, and there is no blood in the urine.

What is it? The issue in scrotal hematomas is whether the testicle is ruptured or not.

Diagnosis. U/S will tell.

Management. If ruptured, surgery will be needed, usually orchiectomy. If intact, only symptomatic treatment.

71. A 41-year-old man presents to the ED reporting that he slipped in the shower and injured his penis. Examination reveals a large penile shaft hematoma with normal appearing glans.

What is it? A classic description of fracture of the tunica albuginea (fracture of the corpora cavernosa)—including the usual cover story given by the patient. These always happen during sexual intercourse, usually with woman on top—but the patient is too embarrassed to explain the true details.

Management. This is a urologic emergency. Prompt surgical repair is needed.

Injury to the Extremities

72. A 25-year-old man is shot with a .22-caliber revolver. The entrance wound is in the anteriolateral aspect of his thigh, and the bullet is seen by x-rays to be embedded in the muscles, posterolateral to the femur.

73. A 25-year-old man is shot with a .22-caliber revolver. The entrance wound is in the anteromedial aspect of his upper thigh, and the exit wound is in the posterolateral aspect of the thigh. He has normal pulses in the leg, and no hematoma at the entrance site. X-rays show the femur to be intact.

74. A 25-year-old man is shot with a .22-caliber revolver. The entrance wound is in the anteromedial aspect of his upper thigh, and the exit wound is in the posterolateral aspect of the thigh. He has a large, expanding hematoma in the upper, inner thigh. The bone is intact.

Apart from the obvious need to fix a bone that might have been shattered by a bullet, the issue in low-velocity gunshot wounds (or stab wounds) of the extremities is the possibility of injury to major vessels. In the first vignette, the anatomy precludes that possibility. Thus the patient only needs cleaning of the wound and tetanus prophylaxis. The bullet can be left where it is.

In the second patient, the anatomy of the area makes vascular injury very likely, and lack of symptoms does not exclude that possibility. At one time, all of these would have been surgically explored. Arteriogram then became the preferred diagnostic modality, and, currently CTA is a highly sensitive non-invasive alternative.

In the third vignette, it is clinically obvious that there is a vascular injury. Surgical exploration is in order. Arteriogram preceding surgical exploration is done only in parts of the body where the very specific site of the vascular injury dictates the use of a particular incision versus another (for instance at the base of the neck and thoracic outlet).

75. A young man is shot through the arm with a .38-caliber revolver. The path of the bullet goes right across the extremity, from medial to lateral sides. He has a large hematoma in the inner aspect of the arm, no distal pulses, radial nerve palsy, and a shattered humerus.

That the patient will need surgery is clear, but the issue here is what to do first. A very delicate vascular repair, and an even more fragile nerve reanastomosis, would be at risk of disruption when the orthopedic surgeons start manipulating, hammering, and screwing the bone. Thus the usual sequence begins with fracture stabilization, then vascular repair (both artery and vein if possible), and last nerve repair. The unavoidable delay in restoring circulation will make a fasciotomy mandatory. Temporary shunting the arterial injury to allow distal perfusion is a good solution if offered as a choice, but is easier said than done in real life.

76. In a hunting accident, a young man is shot in the leg with a high-powered, big-game hunting rifle. He has an entrance wound in the upper outer thigh that is 1 cm in diameter, and an exit wound in the posteromedial aspect of the thigh that is 8 cm in diameter. The femur is shattered.

Even though the major vessels are not in the path of this bullet, this young man will need to go to the OR to have extensive debridement of the injured tissues. High-velocity bullets (military weapons and big-game hunting rifles) produce a cone of destruction.

77. A 6-year-old girl has her hand, forearm, and lower part of the arm crushed in a car accident. The entire upper extremity looks bruised and battered, although pulses are normal and the bones are not broken.

In addition to possible hyperkalemia, crushing injuries lead to 2 concerns: the myoglobinemia–myoglobinuria–acute renal failure issue and the delayed swelling which may lead to a compartment syndrome. For the first, plenty of fluids, osmotic diuretics (mannitol), and alkalinization of the urine help protect the kidney. For the latter, fasciotomy is the answer.

BURNS

1. You get a phone call from a frantic mother. Her 7-year-old girl spilled Drano all over her arms and legs. You can hear the girl screaming in pain in the background.

Management. The point of this question is that chemical injuries—particularly alkalis—need copious, immediate, profuse irrigation. Instruct the mother to do so right at home with tap water, for at least 30 minutes before rushing the girl to the ED. Do not pick an option where you would be "playing chemist," i.e., soak an alkaline burn with an acid or vice versa.

2. While trying to hook up illegally to cable TV, a man comes in contact with a high-tension electrical power line. He gets an entrance burn wound in the upper outer thigh, and an exit burn lower on the same side.

Management. The issue here is that electrical burns are always much bigger than they appear to be. There is deep tissue destruction. The patient will require extensive surgical debridement. There is also another item (more likely to be the point of the question): myoglobinemia, leading to myoglobinuria and to renal failure. Patient needs lots of IV fluids, diuretics (osmotic if given that choice, i.e., mannitol), perhaps alkalinization of the urine.

If asked about other injuries to rule out, they include posterior dislocation of the shoulder and compression fractures of vertebral bodies (from the violent muscle contractions), and late development of cataracts and demyelinization syndromes.

3. A man is rescued by firemen from a burning building. On admission it is noted that he has burns around the mouth and nose, and the inside of his mouth and throat look like the inside of a chimney.

What is it? There are 2 issues here: carbon monoxide poisoning and respiratory burns, i.e., smoke inhalation producing a chemical burn of the tracheobronchial tree. Both will happen with flame burns in an enclosed space. The burns in the face are an additional clue that most patients rarely have in real life but will be mentioned on the exam to point you in that direction.

For the first issue we determine blood levels of carboxyhemoglobin, and put the patient on 100% oxygen (oxygen therapy will shorten the half-life of carboxyhemoglobin). For the second issue, diagnosis can be made with bronchoscopy, but the actual degree of damage—and the need for supportive therapy—is more likely to be revealed by monitoring of blood gases.

Management. Revolves around respiratory support, with intubation and use of a respirator, if needed.

4. A patient has suffered third-degree burns to both of his arms when his shirt caught on fire while lighting the backyard barbecue. The burned areas are dry, white, leathery, anesthetic, and circumferential all around arms and forearms.

What is it? You are meant to recognize the problem posed by circumferential burns: the leathery eschar will not expand, while the area under the burn will develop massive edema, thus circulation will be cut off. (Or in the case of circumferential burns of the chest, breathing will be compromised.) If the fire were in the open space of the backyard, respiratory burn is not an issue.

Management. Compulsive monitoring of Doppler signals of the peripheral pulses and capillary filling. Escharotomies at the bedside at the first sign of compromised circulation. In deeper burns, fasciotomy may also be needed. If the chest wall is involved and respiration impaired, emergent escharotomy is necessary.

5. A toddler is brought to the ED with burns on both of his buttocks. The areas are moist, have blisters, and are exquisitely painful to touch. The parents report that the child accidentally pulled a pot of boiling water over himself.

What is it? Burns, of course. There are several issues. First: how deep. The description is classic for second-degree burns. (Note that in kids third-degree burn is deep bright red, rather than white leathery as in the adult.) How did it really happen? Scalding burns in kids always brings up the possibility of child abuse, particularly if they have the distribution that you would expect if you grabbed the kid by the arms and legs and dunked him in a pot of boiling water.

Management. For the burn is Silvadene (silver sulfadiazine) cream. Management for the social problem requires reporting to authorities for child abuse.

6. An adult man who weighs x kilograms sustains second- and third-degree burns over—whatever. The burns will be depicted in a front-and-back drawing, indicating what is second-degree (moist, blisters, painful) and what is third-degree (white, leathery, anesthetic). The question will be about fluid resuscitation.

The first order of business will be to figure out the percentage of body surface burned. The rule of nines is used. In the adult, the head is 9% of body surface, each arm is 9%, each leg has two 9%s, and the trunk has 4 9%s.

7. An adult who weighs x kilograms has third-degree burns over... (the calculated surface turns out to be >20%). Fluid administration should be started at a rate of what?

If you are simply asked how fast should the infusion start, rather than what is the calculated total for the whole day, the answer is Ringer's lactate (without sugar) at 1,000 ml/h.

8. An adult man who weighs x kilograms has third-degree burns over... (a set of drawings provides the area). How much is the estimated amount of fluid that will be needed for resuscitation?

If asked this way, remember the old Parkland formula:

4 ml of Ringer's lactate (without sugar) per kilogram of body weight, per percentage of burned area (up to 50%) "for the burn," plus about 2L of 5% dextrose in water (D5W) for maintenance

Give one half in the first 8 hours, the second half in the next 16 hours. Day 2 requires about one half of that calculated amount, and is the time when colloids should be given if one elects to use them. By day 3 there should be a brisk diuresis, and no need for further fluid.

Remember that these amounts are only a guess, to be fine-tuned by the actual response of the patient (primarily hourly urinary output). Higher amounts are needed in patients who have respiratory burn, electrical burns, or recent escharotomies.

The use of the formulas is now less frequently done, since physicians typically end up adjusting the rate of fluid administration on the basis of the urinary output after initial resuscitation.

9. After suitable calculations have been made, a 70-kg adult with extensive third degree burns is receiving Ringer's lactate at the calculated rate. In the first 3 hours his urinary output is 15, 22, and 18 ml.

Most experts aim for an hourly urinary output of at least 0.5 ml/kg, or preferably 1 ml/kg body weight per hour. For patients with electrical burns the flow should be even higher (1 to 2 ml/kg per hour); thus by any criteria this patient needs more fluid.

10. After suitable calculations have been made, a 70-kg adult with extensive third degree burns is receiving Ringer's lactate at the calculated rate. In the first 3 hours his urinary output is 325, 240, and 270 ml.

The opposite of the previous vignette. Somebody is trying to drown this poor guy. The calculation was too generous; the rate of administration has to be scaled back.

11. During the first 48 hours after a major burn, a 70-kg patient received vigorous fluid resuscitation and maintained a urinary output between 45 and 110 ml/h. On postburn day 3—after IV fluids have been discontinued—urinary output reaches 270 to 350 ml/h.

This is the expected. Fluid is coming back from the burn area into the circulation. He does not need more IV fluids to replace these losses.

12. An 8-month-old baby who weighs x kilograms is burned over…areas (depicted in a front-and-back drawing). Second-degree burn will look the same as in the adult; third-degree burn will look deep bright red.

In babies the head is bigger and the legs are smaller, thus the head has two 9%s, whereas both legs add up to 3 (rather than 4) 9%s. Proportionally, fluid needs are greater in children than in adults. Therefore:

- If asked for the rate in the first hour, it should be 20 ml/kg.
- If asked for 24-hour calculations, the formula calls for 4 to 6 ml/kg/%.

13. A patient with second- and third-degree burns over 65% of his body surface is undergoing proper fluid resuscitation. The question asks about management for the burned areas, and other supportive care.

First of all, tetanus prophylaxis. Then suitable cleaning, and use of topical agents. The standard one is silver sulfadiazine. If deep penetration is desired (thick eschar, cartilage), mafenide acetate is the choice (do not use everywhere; it hurts and can produce acidosis). Burns near the eyes are covered with triple antibiotic ointment. Pain medication is given IV.

After about 2–3 weeks, grafts will be done to the areas that did not regenerate. After an initial day or two of NG suction, intensive nutritional support is needed (via the gut, high calorie/high nitrogen). Rehabilitation starts on day 1.

14. A 42-year-old woman drops her hot iron on her lap while doing the laundry. She comes in with the shape of the iron clearly delineated on her upper thigh. The area is white, dry, leathery, anesthetic.

What is the issue? A current favorite of burn treatment is the concept of early excision and grafting. After fluid resuscitation, the typical patient with extensive burns spends 2–3 weeks in the hospital consuming thousands of dollars of health care every day, getting topical treatment to the burn areas and intensive nutritional support in preparation for skin grafting.

In very extensive burns there is no alternative. However, less extensive burns can be taken to the OR and excised and grafted on day 1, saving tons of money. You will not be asked on the exam to provide the fine judgment call for the borderline case that might be managed that way (the experts are routinely doing it in burns under 20% and daring to include patients with as much as 40%), but the vignette is a classic one in which the decision is easy: very small and clearly third-degree.

Management. Early excision and grafting.

BITES AND STINGS

1. A 6-year-old child tries to pet a domestic dog while the dog is eating, and the child's hand is bitten by the dog.

This is considered a provoked attack, and as far as rabies is concerned, only observation of the pet is required (for development of signs of rabies). Tetanus prophylaxis and standard wound care is all that is needed for the child. Had the bite been to the face, and thus near the brain, treatment should be started and then discontinued if it is proven to be not necessary.

2. During a hunting trip, a young man is bitten on the leg by a coyote. The animal is captured and brought to the authorities alive.

Observation of a wild animal for behavioral signs of rabies is impractical. But having the animal available will allow it to be killed and the brain examined for signs of rabies, thus hopefully sparing the hunter the necessity of getting vaccinated. Had the bite been to the face, and thus near the brain, treatment should be started and then discontinued if it is proven to be not necessary.

3. While exploring caves in the Texas hill country, a young man is bitten by bats (that promptly fly away).

Now we do not have the animal to examine. Rabies prophylaxis is mandatory (immunoglobulin plus vaccine).

4. During a hunting trip a hunter is bitten in the leg by a snake. His companion, who is an expert outdoorsman, reports that the snake had elliptical eyes, pits behind the nostrils, big fangs, and rattlers in the tail. The patient arrives at the hospital 1 hour after the bite took place. Physical examination shows 2 fang marks about 2 cm apart, and there is no local pain, swelling, or discoloration.

The description of the snake is indeed that of a poisonous rattlesnake, but even when bitten by a poisonous snake, up to 30% of patients are not envenomated. The most reliable signs of envenomation are excruciating local pain, swelling, and discoloration (usually fully developed within 30 minutes)—none of which this man has. Continued observation (about 12 hours) is all that is needed, plus the standard wound care (including tetanus prophylaxis).

5. During a hunting trip, a hunter is bitten in the leg by a snake. His companion, who is an expert outdoorsman, reports that the snake had elliptical eyes, pits behind the nostrils, big fangs, and rattlers in the tail. The patient arrives at the hospital 1 hour after the bite took place. Physical examination shows two fang marks about 2 cm apart, as well as local edema and ecchymotic discoloration. The area is very painful and tender to palpation.

This patient is envenomated. Blood should be drawn for typing and crossmatch, coagulation studies, and renal and liver function. The mainstay of therapy is antivenin, of which several vials have to be given. The product currently preferred is CroFab. Surgical excision of the bite site and fasciotomy are only needed in extremely severe cases.

6. While playing in the backyard of her south Texas home, a 6-year-old girl is bitten by a rattlesnake. At the time of hospital admission she has severe signs of envenomation.

The point of this vignette is to remind you that snake antivenin is one of the very few medicines for which the dose is *not* calculated on the basis of the size of the patient. The dose of antivenin depends on the *amount of venom injected*, regardless of the size and age of the victim.

7. During a picnic outing, a young girl inadvertently bumps into a beehive and is stung repeatedly by angry bees. She is seen 20 minutes later and found to be wheezing, hypotensive, and madly scratching an urticarial rash.

Epinephrine is the drug of choice (0.3 to 0.5 ml of 1:1000 solution). The stingers have to be carefully removed.

8. While rummaging around her attic, a woman is bitten by a spider that she describes as black, with a red hourglass mark in her belly. The patient has nausea and vomiting and severe generalized muscle cramps.

Black widow spider bite. The antidote is IV calcium gluconate. Muscle relaxants also help.

9. A patient seeks help for a very painful ulceration that he discovered in his forearm on arising this morning. Yesterday he spent several hours cleaning up the attic, and he thinks he may have been "bitten by a bug." The ulcer is 1 cm in diameter, with a necrotic center with a surrounding halo of erythema.

Probably a brown recluse spider bite. Dapsone will help. Local excision and skin grafting may be needed. All necrotic tissue must be debrided/excised.

10. A 22-year-old gang leader comes to the ED with a small, 1-cm deep sharp cut over the knuckle of the right middle finger. He says he cut himself with a screwdriver while fixing his car.

What is it? The description is classic for a human bite. No, nobody actually bit him—he did it by punching someone in the mouth and getting cut with the teeth that were smashed by his fist. The imaginative cover story usually comes with this kind of lesion. The point of management is that human bites are bacteriologically the dirtiest that one can get and antibiotics are given. Rabies shots will not be needed, but surgical exploration by an orthopedic surgeon will be required as well as antibiotics.

PEDIATRIC ORTHOPEDICS

1. In the newborn nursery it is noted that a child has uneven gluteal folds. Physical examination of the hips reveals that one of them can be easily dislocated posteriorly with a jerk and a "click," and returned to normal position with a "snapping." The family is concerned because a previous child had the same problem.

What is it? Developmental dysplasia of the hip (congenital dislocation of the hip)

Diagnosis. The physical examination should suffice, but if there is any doubt, do a sonogram.

Management. Abduction splinting with Pavlik harness

2. A 6-year-old boy has insidious development of limping with decreased hip motion. He complains occasionally of knee pain on that side. He walks into the office with an antalgic gait. Passive motion of the hip is guarded.

What is it? In this age group, Legg-Calve-Perthes disease (avascular necrosis of the capital femoral epiphysis). Remember that hip pathology can show up with knee pain. Management is AP and lateral x-rays for diagnosis. Contain the femoral head within the acetabulum by casting and crutches.

3. A 13-year-old obese boy complains of pain in the groin (it could be the knee) and is noted by the family to be limping. He sits in the office with the sole of the foot on the affected side pointing toward the other foot. Physical examination is normal for the knee, but shows limited hip motion. As the hip is flexed, the leg goes into external rotation and cannot be rotated internally.

What is it? Forget the details: a bad hip in this age group is slipped capital femoral epiphysis, an orthopedic emergency. Management is AP and lateral x-rays for diagnosis. The orthopedic surgeons will pin the femoral head in place.

4. A young toddler has had the flu for several days, but until 2 days ago he was walking around normally. He now absolutely refuses to move one of his legs. He is in pain and holds the leg with the hip flexed, in slight abduction and external rotation, and you cannot examine that hip—he will not let you move it. He has elevated sedimentation rate.

What is it? Another orthopedic emergency: septic hip. Aspiration of the hip under general anesthesia to confirm the diagnosis, and open arthrotomy is performed for drainage.

5. A child with a febrile illness but no history of trauma has persistent, severe localized pain in a bone.

What is it? Acute hematogenous osteomyelitis. X-ray will not show anything for 2 weeks. MRI is diagnostic. Then give antibiotics.

6. A 2-year-old child is brought in by concerned parents because he is bowlegged.

7. A 5-year-old child is brought in by concerned parents because he is knockkneed.

Genu varum (bow-leg) is normal up to age 3. Genu valgus (knock-knee) is normal ages 4–8. Thus, neither of these children needs therapy. Should the varum deformity (bow-legs) persist beyond its normal age range, i.e., age >3, Blount disease is the most common problem (a disturbance of the medial proximal tibial growth plate). In that case, surgery can be performed.

8. A 14-year-old boy says he injured his knee while playing football. Although there is no swelling of the knee joint, he complains of persistent pain right over the tibial tubercle, which is aggravated by contraction of the quadriceps. Physical examination shows localized tenderness right over the tibial tubercle.

This is another one with a fancy name: Osgood-Schlatter disease (osteochondrosis of the tibial tubercle). It is usually treated with immobilization of the knee in an extension or cylinder cast for 4–6 weeks, if more conservative management fails (rest, ice, compression, and elevation).

9. A baby boy is born with both feet turned inward. Physical examination shows that there is plantar flexion of the ankle, inversion of the foot, adduction of the forefoot, and internal rotation of the tibia.

This is the complex deformity known as club foot (fancy name: talipes equinovarus). The child needs serial plaster casts started in the neonatal period. The sequence of correction starts with the adducted forefoot, then the hindfoot varus, and finally the equinus. About 50% of patients respond completely and need no surgery; those who require surgery are operated on age >6–8 months, but <1–2 years.

10. A 12-year-old girl is referred by the school nurse because of potential scoliosis.

The thoracic spine is curved toward the right, and when the girl bends forward a "hump" is noted over her right thorax. The patient has not yet started to menstruate.

Management. This is too complicated for the exam, but the point is that scoliosis may progress until skeletal maturity is reached. Baseline x-rays are needed to monitor progression. At the onset of menses skeletal maturity is ~80%, so this patient still has a way to go. Bracing may be needed to arrest progression. Pulmonary function could be limited if there is large deformity.

Fractures

11. A 4-year-old falls down the stairs and fractures his humerus. He is placed in a cast at the nearby "doc in the box," and he is seen by his regular pediatrician 2 days later. At that time he seems to be doing fine, but AP and lateral x-rays show significant angulation of the broken bone.

Nothing else is needed. Except for rotational deformities, children have such tremendous ability to heal and remodel broken bones that almost any reasonable alignment and immobilization will end up with a good result. In fact, fractures in children are no big deal—with a few exceptions that are illustrated in the next few vignettes.

12. An 8-year-old boy falls on his right hand with the arm extended, and he breaks his elbow by hyperextension. X-rays show a supracondylar fracture of the humerus. The distal fragment is displaced posteriorly.

This type of fracture is common in children, but it is important because it may produce vascular or nerve injuries—or both—and end up with a Volkmann contracture. Although it can usually be treated with appropriate casting or traction (and rarely needs surgery), the answer revolves around careful monitoring of vascular and nerve integrity, and vigilance regarding development of a compartment syndrome.

13. A child sustains a fracture of a long bone, involving the epiphyses and growth plate. The epiphyses and growth plate are laterally displaced from the metaphyses, but they are in one piece, i.e., the fracture does not cross the epiphyses or growth plate and does not involve the joint.

14. A child sustains a fracture of a long bone that extends through the joint, the epiphyses, the growth plate, and a piece of the metaphyses.

In the first example, even though the dreaded growth plate is involved it has not been divided by the fracture. Treatment by closed reduction is sufficient.

In the second example, there are 2 pieces of growth plate. Unless they are very precisely aligned, growth will be disturbed. Open reduction and internal fixation will be needed.

ADULT ORTHOPEDICS

1. A man who fell from a second floor window has clinical evidence of fracture of his femur. The vignette gives you a choice of x-rays to order.

Here are the rules:

- Always get x-rays at 90° to each other (for instance, AP and lateral).
- Always include the joints above and below.
- If appropriate (this case is), check the other bones that might be in the same line of force (here, the lumbar spine).

2. While playing football, a college student fractures his clavicle. The point of tenderness is at the junction of the middle and distal thirds of the clavicle.

Place the arm in a sling or figure of 8 splint. Young women may request fixation by surgery, to achieve a better cosmetic result.

3. A 55-year-old woman falls in the shower and hurts her right shoulder. She shows up in the ED with her arm held close to her body, but rotated outward as if she were going to shake hands. She is in pain and will not move the arm from that position. There is numbness in a small area of her shoulder, over the deltoid muscle.

What is it? Anterior dislocation of the shoulder, with axillary nerve damage.

Management. Get AP and lateral x-rays for diagnosis. Reduce.

4. After a grand mal seizure, a 32-year-old epileptic notices pain in her right shoulder, and she cannot move it. She goes to the nearby "doc in a box," where she has x-rays and is diagnosed as having a sprain and given pain medication. The next day she still has the same pain and inability to move the arm. She comes to the ED with the arm held close to her body, in a normal (i.e., not externally rotated, but internally rotated) protective position.

What is it? Posterior dislocation of the shoulder. Very easy to miss on regular x-rays.

Management. Get x-rays again but order axillary view or scapular lateral.

5. An elderly woman with osteoporosis falls on her outstretched hand. She comes in with a deformed and painful wrist that looks like a "dinner fork." X-rays show a dorsally displaced, dorsally angulated fracture of the distal radius and small, nondisplaced fracture of the ulnar stylus.

This is the famous Colles' fracture. It is treated with close reduction and long arm cast.

6. During a rowdy demonstration and police crackdown, a young man is hit with a nightstick on his outer forearm that he had raised to protect himself. He is found to have a diaphyseal fracture of the proximal ulna, with anterior dislocation of the radial head.

Another classic with a fancy name: Monteggia fracture. The patient needs closed reduction of the radial head, and possible open reduction and internal fixation of the ulnar fracture.

7. Another victim of the same melee has a fracture of the distal third of the radius and dorsal dislocation of the distal radioulnar joint.

This one is Galeazzi fracture and is quite similar to Monteggia in terms of the resultant instability. The fractured radius may need open reduction and internal fixation, while the dislocated joint may be manipulated back into proper position and casted in supination.

8. A young adult falls on an outstretched hand and comes in complaining of wrist pain. On physical examination, he is distinctly tender to palpation over the anatomic snuff-box. AP and lateral x-rays are read as negative.

Another classic, this is a fracture of the scaphoid bone (carpal navicular). These are notorious because x-rays will not show them for 2–3 weeks, and they have a high rate of nonunion. The history and physical findings (the tenderness in the snuff-box) are sufficient to indicate the use of a thumb spica cast, with repeat x-rays 3 weeks later.

9. A young adult falls on an outstretched hand and comes in complaining of wrist pain. On physical examination he is distinctly tender to palpation over the anatomic snuff-box. AP, lateral, and oblique x-rays show a displaced and angulated fracture of the scaphoid.

Displaced and angulated; will need open reduction and internal fixation.

10. During a barroom fight, a young man throws a punch at somebody, but misses and ends up hitting the wall. He comes in with a swollen and tender right hand. X-rays show fracture of the fourth and fifth metacarpal necks.

Metacarpal necks, typically the fourth or the fifth (or both), take the brunt of one's anger when trying to hit somebody but miss. Treatment depends on the degree of angulation, displacement, or rotary malalignment. Closed reduction and ulnar gutter splint for the mild ones, Kirschner-wire or plate fixation for the bad ones.

11. A 77-year-old man falls in the nursing home and hurts his hip. He shows up with the affected leg shortened and externally rotated. X-rays show that he has a displaced femoral neck fracture.

The point of this vignette is that blood supply to the femoral head is compromised in this setting, and the patient is better off with a metal prosthesis put in, rather than an attempt at fixing the bone.

12. A 77-year-old man falls in the nursing home and hurts his hip. He shows up with the affected leg shortened and externally rotated. X-rays show that he has an intertrochanteric fracture.

These can be fixed with less concern about avascular necrosis. Open reduction and pinning are usually performed. Immobilization in these old people often leads to deep venous thrombosis and pulmonary embolus; thus an additional choice for postoperative anticoagulation may be offered in the question.

13. The unrestrained front-seat passenger in a car that crashes sustains a closed fracture of the femoral shaft.

There are many ways to deal with fractured femurs, but intramedullary rod fixation is commonly done.

14. The unrestrained front-seat passenger in a car that crashes sustains closed comminuted fractures of both femoral shafts. Shortly after admission, he develops BP 80/50 mm Hg, pulse 110/min, and venous pressure 0. The remainder of the physical examination and x-ray survey (chest, pelvis) are unremarkable. Sonogram of the abdomen done in the ED was negative.

This is a throwback to the trauma vignettes to remind you that femur fractures may bleed into the tissues sufficiently to cause hypovolemic shock. Fixation will diminish the blood loss, and fluid resuscitation and blood transfusions will take care of the shock.

15. The unrestrained front-seat passenger in a car that crashes sustains closed comminuted fractures of both femoral shafts. Twelve hours after admission, he develops disorientation, fever, and scleral petechia. Dyspnea is evident shortly thereafter, at which time blood gases show Po2 of 60.

Another repeated topic: fat embolism. Respiratory support is the centerpiece of the treatment.

16. A college student is tackled while playing football, and he develops severe knee pain. When examined shortly thereafter, the knee is swollen, and he has pain on direct palpation over the medial aspect of the knee. With the knee flexed at 30°, passive abduction elicits pain in the same area, and the leg can be abducted further out than the normal, contralateral leg (valgus stress test).

17. A college student is tackled while playing football, and he develops severe knee pain. When examined shortly thereafter, the knee is swollen, and he has pain on direct palpation over the lateral aspect of the knee. With the knee flexed at 30°, passive adduction elicits pain in the same area, and the leg can be adducted further out than the normal, contralateral leg (varus stress test).

The medial collateral ligament is injured in the first example, whereas the second example depicts an injury to the lateral collateral ligament. A hinged cast is the usual treatment for either isolated injury. When several ligaments are torn, surgical repair is preferred.

18. A college student is tackled while playing football, and he develops severe knee swelling and pain. On physical examination with the knee flexed at 90°, the leg can be pulled anteriorly, like a drawer being opened. A similar finding can be elicited with the knee fixed at 20° by grasping the thigh with one hand, and pulling the leg with the other.

This is a lesion of the anterior cruciate ligament, shown by the anterior drawer test and the Lachman test. Further definition of the extent of internal knee injuries can be done with MRI.

Sedentary patients may be treated just with immobilization and rehabilitation, but athletes require arthroscopic reconstruction.

19. A college athlete injured his knee while playing basketball. He has been to several physicians who have prescribed pain medication and a variety of splints and bandages, but he still has a swollen knee and knee pain. He describes catching and locking that limit his knee motion, and he swears that when his knee is forcefully extended there is a "click" in the joint. He has been told that his x-rays are normal.

Meniscal tears may be difficult to diagnose clinically, but MRI will show them beautifully. Arthroscopic repair is done, trying to save as much of the meniscus as possible. If complete meniscectomy is done, late degenerative arthritis will ensue. Some orthopedic surgeons prefer to repair meniscal injuries with an open operation.

20. A young recruit complains of localized pain in his tibia after a forced march at boot camp. He is tender to palpation over a very specific point on the bone, but x-rays are normal.

What is it? Stress fracture. The lesson here is that stress fractures will not show up radiologically until 2 weeks later. Treat as if he has a fracture (cast) and repeat the x-ray in 2 weeks. Non–weight bearing (crutches) is another option.

21. A pedestrian is hit by a car. Physical examination shows the leg to be angulated midway between the knee and the ankle. X-rays confirm fractures of the shaft of the tibia and fibula.

Casting takes care of the ones that can be easily reduced. Intramedullary nailing is needed for the ones that cannot be aligned.

22. A pedestrian is hit by a car. Physical examination shows the leg to be angulated midway between the knee and the ankle. X-rays confirm fractures of the shaft of the tibia and fibula. Satisfactory alignment is achieved, and a long leg cast applied. In the ensuing 8 hours the patient complains of increasing pain. When the cast is removed, the pain persists, the muscle compartments feel tight, and there is excruciating pain with passive extension of the toes.

Compartment syndrome is a distinct hazard after fractures of the leg (the forearm and the lower leg are the two places with the highest incidence of compartment syndrome). Fasciotomy is needed here.

23. An out-of-shape, recently divorced 42-year-old man is trying to impress a young woman by challenging her to a game of tennis. In the middle of the game, a loud "pop" is heard (like a gunshot), and the man falls to the ground clutching his ankle. He limps off the courts, with pain and swelling in the back of the lower leg, but still able to dorsiflex his foot. When he seeks medical help the next day, palpation of his Achilles tendon reveals an obvious defect right beneath the skin.

This is a classic presentation for rupture of the Achilles tendon. Casting in equinus position will allow healing after several months, or open surgical repair may do it sooner.

24. While running to catch a bus, an old man twists his ankle and falls on his inverted foot. AP, lateral, and mortise X-rays show displaced fractures of both malleoli.

A very common injury. When the foot is forcefully rotated (in either direction), the talus pushes and breaks one malleolus and pulls off the other one. Open reduction and internal fixation is needed in this case because the fragments are displaced.

Orthopedic Emergencies

25. A middle-aged homeless man is brought to the ED because of very severe pain in his forearm. He passed out after drinking a bottle of cheap wine and fell asleep on a park bench for an indeterminate time, probably over 12 hours. There are no signs of trauma, but the muscles in his forearm are very firm and tender to palpation. Passive motion of his fingers and wrist elicit excruciating pain. Pulses at the wrist are normal.

Classic compartment syndrome. Emergency fasciotomy is needed. Note that normal pulses do not rule out this diagnosis.

26. A patient presents to the ED complaining of moderate but persistent pain in his leg under a long leg plaster cast that was applied 6 hours earlier for a fracture.

The point of this vignette is that you do not do anything for pain under a cast, not even pain medication. The cast must be removed right away. It may be too tight, it may be compromising blood supply, or it may have rubbed off a piece of skin. Your only acceptable option is to remove the cast.

27. A young man involved in a motorcycle accident has an obvious open (compound) fracture of his right thigh. The femur is sticking out through a jagged skin laceration.

An open fracture is an orthopedic emergency. This patient may need to have other problems treated first (abdominal bleeding, intracranial hematomas, chest tubes, etc.), but the open fracture should be in the OR getting cleaned and reduced within 6 hours of the injury.

28. A front-seat passenger in a car that had a head-on collision relates that he hit the dashboard with his knees, and complains of pain in the right hip. He lies in the stretcher in the ED with the right lower extremity shortened, adducted, and internally rotated.

What is it? Another orthopedic emergency: posterior dislocation of the hip. The blood supply of the femoral head is tenuous, and delay in reduction could lead to avascular necrosis.

Management. X-rays and emergency reduction.

29. A healthy 24-year-old man steps on a rusty nail at the stables where he works as a horse breeder. Three days later he is brought to the ED moribund, with a swollen, dusky foot, in which one can feel gas crepitation.

What is it? Gas gangrene. Management is a lot of IV penicillin and immediate surgical debridement of dead tissue, followed by a trip to the nearest hyperbaric chamber for hyperbaric oxygen treatment.

30. A 48-year-old man breaks his arm when he falls down the stairs. X-rays demonstrate an oblique fracture of the middle to distal thirds of the humerus. Physical examination shows that he cannot dorsiflex (extend) his wrist.

Fractures of the humeral shaft can injure the radial nerve, which courses in a spiral groove right around the posterior aspect of that bone. However, surgical exploration is not usually needed. Hanging arm cast or coaptation splint are used, and the nerve function returns eventually. However, if the nerve was okay when the patient came in, and becomes paralyzed after closed reduction of the bone, the nerve is entrapped and surgery has to be performed.

31. A football player is hit straight on his right leg, and he suffers a posterior dislocation of his knee.

The point here is that posterior dislocation of the knee can nail the popliteal artery. Attention to integrity of pulses, Doppler studies or CT angio, and prompt reduction are the key issues.

32. A window cleaner falls from a third-story scaffold and lands on his feet. Physical examination and x-rays show comminuted fractures of both calcanei.

Compression fractures of the thoracic or lumbar spine are the associated, hidden injuries that have to be looked for in this case.

33. In a head-on automobile collision, the unrestrained front-seat passenger strikes the dashboard and windshield. He comes in with facial lacerations, upper extremity fractures, and blunt trauma to his chest and abdomen.

In the confusion of dealing with multiple traumas, it is possible to miss less-obvious injuries. In this scenario, as the knees strike the dashboard, the femoral heads may drive backward into the pelvis, or out of the acetabulum.

34. The unrestrained front-seat passenger in a car that crashes at high speed is brought into the ED with multiple facial fractures and a closed head injury.

The ultimate hidden injury (because of the devastating complications if missed) is the fracture of the cervical spine. A CT scan must be done to rule it out.

Common Hand Problems

35. A 43-year-old secretary who types a lot at work complains about numbness and tingling in the hand, particularly at night. On physical examination, when asked to hang her hand limply in front of her, numbness and tingling are reproduced over the distribution of the median nerve (the radial side 3 1/2 fingers). The same happens when her median nerve is pressed over the carpal tunnel, or when it is percussed.

Carpal tunnel syndrome is diagnosed clinically, and this vignette is typical. The American Academy of Orthopedic Surgery recommends that wrist x-rays (including carpal tunnel view) be done, primarily to rule out other things. Initial treatment is splints and anti-inflammatories. If surgery is needed, electromyography and nerve conduction velocity should precede it.

36. A 58-year-old woman describes that she awakens at night with her right middle finger acutely flexed, and she is unable to extend it. She can do it only by pulling on it with her other hand, at which time she feels a painful "snap."

This is trigger finger. Steroid injections are tried first, and surgery is performed if needed.

37. A young mother complains of pain along the radial side of the wrist and the first dorsal compartment. She relates that the pain is often caused by the position of wrist flexion and simultaneous thumb extension that she assumes to carry the head of her baby. On physical examination the pain is reproduced by asking her to hold her thumb inside her closed fist, and then forcing the wrist into ulnar deviation.

De Quervain tenosynovitis. Splints and antiinflammatories can help, but steroid injection is best. Surgery is rarely needed.

38. A 72-year-old man of Norwegian ancestry has a contracted hand that can no longer be extended and be placed flat on a table. Palmar fascial nodules can be felt.

Dupuytren contracture. Surgery may be needed.

39. A 33-year-old carpenter accidentally drives a small nail into the pulp of his index finger, but he pays no attention to the injury at the time. Two days later he shows up in the ER, with throbbing pulp pain, fever, and all the signs of an abscess within the pulp of the affected finger.

This kind of abscess is called a *felon*, and like all abscesses it has to be drained. There is an urgency to it, however, because the pulp is a closed space and the process is equivalent to a compartment syndrome.

40. A young man falls while skiing, and as he does he jams his thumb into the snow. Physical examination shows collateral laxity at the thumb metacarpophalangeal joint.

This one is "gamekeeper's thumb." The injury was to the ulnar collateral ligament of the thumb. If not treated it can be dysfunctional and painful, and can lead to arthritis. Casting is usually done.

41. Two thieves grab a woman's purse and run away with it. She tries to grab one of the offenders by his jacket, but he pulls away, hurting the woman's hand in the process. Now, when she makes a fist, the distal phalanx of her ring finger does not flex with the others.

42. While playing volleyball, a young woman injures her middle finger. She cannot extend the distal phalanx.

Two classic tendon injuries, with appropriate names: jersey finger (to the flexor), and mallet finger (to the extensor). Splinting is usually the first line of treatment.

43. While working at a bookbinding shop, a young man suffers a traumatic amputation of his index finger. The finger was cleanly severed at its base.

Replantation of severed digits is no longer "miracle surgery." It is commonly done at specialized centers, and regular physicians should know how to handle the amputated part. The answer is to clean it with sterile saline, wrap it in saline-moistened gauze, place it in a plastic bag, and place the bag on a bed of ice.

The digit should not be placed in antiseptic solutions or alcohol, put in dry ice, or allowed to freeze.

Back Pain

44. A 45-year-old man complains of aching back pain for several months. He was told previously that he had muscle spasms, and was given analgesics and muscle relaxants. He comes in now because of the sudden onset of very severe back pain that came on when he tried to lift a heavy object. The pain is like an electrical shock that shoots down his leg; it is aggravated by sneezing, coughing, and straining, and it prevents him from ambulating. He keeps the affected leg flexed. Straight leg-raising gives excruciating pain.

What is it? Lumbar disk herniation. Peak age incidence is in age 40s, and virtually all those cases are at L4–L5 or L5–S1.

- If the "lightning" exits the foot by the big toe, it is L4–L5.
- If the "lightning" exits by the little toe, it is L5–S1.

Management is MRI for diagnosis. Bed rest and pain control will take care of most of these. Use neurosurgical intervention only if there is progressive weakness or sphincteric deficits.

45. A 46-year-old man has sudden onset of very severe back pain that came on when he tried to lift a heavy object. The pain is like an electrical shock that shoots down his leg, and it prevents him from ambulating. He keeps the affected leg flexed. Straight leg-raising test gives excruciating pain. He has a distended bladder, flaccid rectal sphincter, and perineal saddle area anesthesia.

The cauda equina syndrome is a surgical emergency.

46. A young man began to have chronic back pain at age 34. Pain and stiffness have been progressive. He describes morning stiffness, and pain that is worse at rest, but improves with activity. Two years ago, he was treated for uveitis.

Think ankylosing spondylitis. X-rays will eventually show "bamboo spine." Antiinflammatory agents and physical therapy are used.

47. A 72-year-old man has had a 20-pound weight loss, and he complains of low back pain. The pain is worse at night and is unrelieved by rest or positional changes.

Suggestive of metastatic malignancy. If advanced, x-rays will show it. At a higher cost, an MRI will make a reliable, early diagnosis.

Leg Ulcers

48. A 67-year-old diabetic has an indolent, unhealing ulcer at the heel of the foot.

What is it? Ulcer at a pressure point in a diabetic is caused by neuropathy. Once it has happened, it is unlikely to heal because the microcirculation is poor also. The infection would be osteomyelitis.

Management is to control the diabetes, keep the ulcer clean, keep the leg elevated, and be resigned to the idea that the foot may need to be amputated. The other common location is the first metatarsophalangeal joint.

49. A 67-year-old smoker with high cholesterol and coronary disease has an indolent, unhealing ulcer at the tip of his toe. The toe is blue, and he has no peripheral pulses in that extremity.

What is it? Ischemic ulcers are at the farthest away point from where the blood comes.

Management. Doppler studies looking for pressure gradient, MRI angio or CT angio. Lack of pulses is concerning for an inherent vascular problem; revascularization (i.e. stenting or surgical bypass) may be possible, and then the ulcer may heal.

50. A 44-year-old obese woman has an indolent, unhealing ulcer above her right medial malleolus. The skin around it is thick and hyperpigmented. She has frequent episodes of cellulitis, and has varicose veins.

What is it? Venous stasis ulcer.

Management. Duplex scanning, Unna boot, support stockings. Varicose vein surgery or endoluminal ablation may ultimately be needed.

51. A 40-year-old man has had a chronic draining sinus in his lower leg since he had an episode of osteomyelitis at age 12. In the last few months he has developed an indolent, dirty-looking ulcer at the site, with "heaped up" tissue growth at the edges.

52. Ever since she had an untreated third-degree burn to her lower leg at age 14, a 38-year-old immigrant from Latin America has had shallow ulcerations at the scar site that heal and break down all the time. In the last few months she has developed an indolent, dirty-looking ulcer at the site, with "heaped up" tissue growth around the edges, which is steadily growing and shows no sign of healing.

Both of these are classic vignettes for the development of squamous cell carcinoma at long-standing, chronic irritation sites. The name Marjolin ulcer has been applied to these tumors. Obviously biopsy is the first diagnostic step, and wide local excision (with subsequent skin grafting) is the appropriate therapy.

Foot Pain

53. An older, overweight man complains of disabling, sharp heel pain every time his foot strikes the ground. The pain is worse in the mornings, preventing him from putting any weight on the heel. X-rays show a bony spur matching the location of his pain, and physical examination shows exquisite tenderness right over that heel spur.

Although all the signs point to that bony spur as the culprit, this is in fact plantar fasciitis—a very common but poorly understood problem that needs symptomatic treatment until it resolves spontaneously within 12 to 18 months. Podiatrists often remove the spur anyway; although the spur is not the initial problem, its removal can accelerate recovery.

54. A woman who usually wears high-heeled, pointed shoes complains of pain in the forefoot after prolonged standing or walking. Physical examination shows a very tender spot in the third interspace, between the third and fourth toes.

This one is a Morton neuroma, which is an inflammation of the common digital nerve. If conservative management (more-sensible shoes, among other things) does not suffice, the neuroma may be excised.

55. A 55-year-old obese man suddenly develops swelling, redness, and exquisite pain at the first metatarsal–phalangeal joints.

Gout. The diagnosis of the acute attack is done with identification of uric acid crystals in fluid from the joint. Treatment of the acute attack relies on indomethacin and colchicine. Long-term control of serum uric acid levels is done with allopurinol or probenecid.

TUMORS

1. A 16-year-old boy complains of low-grade but constant pain in the distal femur present for several months. He has local tenderness in the area, but is otherwise asymptomatic. X-rays show a large bone tumor breaking through the cortex into the adjacent soft tissues and exhibiting a "sunburst" pattern.

2. A 10-year-old complains of persistent pain deep in the middle of the thigh. X-rays show a large, fusiform bone tumor, pushing the cortex out and producing periosteal "onion skinning."

Primary malignant bone tumors are also diseases of young people. Our vignettes illustrate each of these, but this is such a specialized field that you may just be asked to diagnose "malignant bone tumor" without picking the specific kind.

*   Most common: osteogenic sarcoma
    *   Seen in ages 10–25
    *   Usually occurs around the knee (lower femur or upper tibia)
*   Second-most common: Ewing's sarcoma
    *   Seen in younger children (ages 5–15)
    *   Grows in the diaphyses of long bones

Management. Do not mess with these and do not attempt biopsy. Referral is needed, both to an orthopedic surgeon (every 3 years) and to a specialist on bone tumors.

3. A 66-year-old woman picks up a bag of groceries, and her arm snaps broken.

What is it? A pathologic fracture (i.e., for trivial reasons) means bone tumor, which in the vast majority of cases will be metastatic. Get x-rays to diagnose this particular broken bone, whole body bone scans to identify other metastases, and start looking for the primary. In women, it is the breast (lytic bone lesions). In men, it is the prostate. Lung is second most common in both men and women.

4. A 60-year-old man complains of fatigue and pain at specific places on several bones. He is found to be anemic, and x-rays show multiple punched out lytic lesions throughout the skeleton.

Multiple lytic lesions in an old anemic man suggest multiple myeloma. X-rays are diagnostic, and additional tests include Bence-Jones protein in the urine and abnormal immunoglobulins in the blood. The latter are detectable by serum electrophoresis and better yet by immuno-electrophoresis.

Management. Chemotherapy is the usual treatment. Thalidomide is used for refractory cases.

5. A 58-year-old woman has a soft tissue tumor in her thigh. It has been growing steadily for 6 months. It is located deep into the thigh, is firm, is fixed to surrounding structures, and measures ~8 cm in diameter.

What is it? Soft tissue sarcoma is the concern.

Diagnosis. Start with MRI. Leave biopsy and further management to the experts.

PREOPERATIVE ASSESSMENT

Cardiac Risk

1. A 72-year-old man with a history of multiple myocardial infarctions is scheduled to have an elective sigmoid resection for diverticular disease. A preoperative radionuclide ventriculography shows an ejection fraction <0.35.

This is a "no-go" situation in which cardiac risk in noncardiac surgery is prohibitive. With this ejection fraction, the incidence of perioperative MI is 75–85%, and the mortality for such an event is around 55–90%. Probably the only option here is not to operate, but to continue with medical therapy for the diverticular disease. Should he develop an abscess, percutaneous drainage would be the only possible intervention.

2. A 72-year-old chronically bedridden man is being considered for emergency cholecystectomy for acute cholecystitis that is not responding to medical management. He had a transmural MI 4 months ago, and currently has atrial fibrillation, 8–10 premature ventricular beats/min, and jugular venous distention.

This patient is a compendium of almost all of the items that Goldman has compiled as predictors of operative cardiac risk. In fact he adds up to 50 points, and anything >25 points (class IV) gives a mortality in excess of 22%. Here again the best option would be to treat the cholecystitis in a different way (percutaneous cholecystostomy tube being the obvious choice).

3. A 72-year-old man is scheduled to have an elective sigmoid resection for diverticular disease. In the preoperative evaluation it is noted that he has venous jugular distention.

Now we have fewer items, but CHF is the worst one on the list (the other one here is his age). The failure has to be treated first, with ACE inhibitors, beta-blockers, digitalis, and diuretics.

4. A 72-year-old man is scheduled to have an elective sigmoid resection for diverticular disease. In the preoperative evaluation it is ascertained that he had a transmural MI 2 months ago.

The next worst Goldman finding is the recent MI (<6 months). Time is the best therapy for that one. Mortality is highest within 3 months of the MI (near 40%), but is brought down considerably >6 months (6%). Waiting is the obvious choice here. If our hand is forced and earlier operation becomes mandatory, admission to the ICU the day before surgery is recommended, to "optimize" all the cardiac parameters.

5. A 72-year-old man who needs to have elective repair of a large abdominal aortic aneurysm has a history of severe, progressive angina.

For many years it was believed that coronary revascularization prior to major surgery improved the risk of the latter. Current reviews of the available evidence suggest that it does not. The planned surgery for the aneurysm can be done first if it is more urgent than addressing the angina.

Pulmonary Risk

6. A 61-year-old man with a 60 pack-year smoking history and physical evidence of chronic obstructive pulmonary disease (COPD) needs elective surgical repair of an abdominal aortic aneurysm. He currently smokes 1 pack per day.

Smoking is by far the most common cause of increased pulmonary risk, and the main problem is compromised ventilation (high Pco2 and low FEV1) rather than compromised oxygenation. Start the evaluation with FEV1. If it is abnormal, perform blood gases. Cessation of smoking for 8 weeks and intensive respiratory therapy (physical therapy, expectorants, incentive spirometry, humidified air) should precede surgery.

Hepatic Risk

7. A cirrhotic is bleeding from a duodenal ulcer. Surgical intervention is being considered. His bilirubin is 3.5, prothrombin time 22 seconds, and serum albumin 2.5. He has ascites and encephalopathy.

Please don't! Any one of those items alone (bilirubin >2, albumin <3, prothrombin >16, and encephalopathy) predicts a mortality >40%. If 3 of them are present, the number is 85%. If all 4 are present, the number is 100%.

8. A cirrhotic with a blood ammonia concentration >150 ng/dl needs an operation.

9. A cirrhotic with an albumin level <2 needs an operation.

10. A cirrhotic with a bilirubin >4 needs an operation.

Another way to look at liver risk is to see if any one of the previously listed findings is deranged to an even greater degree. Any one of these 3 examples would carry a mortality of about 80%. A deranged prothrombin time is slightly kinder to the patient, predicting only 40–60% mortality. Death, incidentally, occurs with high-output cardiac failure with low peripheral resistance.

Nutritional Risk

11. An elderly gentleman needs palliative surgery for an advanced cancer of the colon. He has lost 20% of his body weight over the past 2 months, and his serum albumin is 2.7. Further testing reveals anergy to injected skin-test antigens and a serum transferrin level <200 mg/dl.

Any one of these 4 findings indicates severe nutritional depletion. All 4 leave no doubt as to the enormous operative risk that this man represents. Surprisingly, as few as 4–5 days of preoperative nutritional support (preferably via the gut) can make a big difference, and 7–10 days would be optimal if there is no big hurry to operate.

Metabolic Risk

12. An elderly diabetic man presents with a clinical picture of acute cholecystitis that has been present for 3 days. He is profoundly dehydrated, in coma, and has blood sugar 950, severe acidosis, and ketone bodies "all over the place."

The treatment of diabetes is not within the scope of this surgical review, but we should point out that someone in overt diabetic ketoacidotic coma is not a surgical candidate, no matter how urgent the operation might be. The metabolic problem has to be addressed first in this case (although aiming for complete correction to normal values would be unrealistic as long as that rotten gallbladder is there). Temporization of the cholecystitis can be achieved with a percutaneous cholecystostomy tube with cholecystectomy performed when acidosis has resolved.

POSTOPERATIVE COMPLICATIONS

Fever

1. Shortly after the onset of a general anesthetic with inhaled halothane and muscle relaxation with succinylcholine, a patient develops a rapid rise in body temperature, exceeding 104° F. Metabolic acidosis and hypercalcemia are also noted. A family member died under general anesthesia several years before, but no details are available.

A classic case of malignant hyperthermia. The history should have been a warning, but once the problem develops, treat with IV dantrolene plus the obvious support measures: 100% oxygen, correction of the acidosis, and cooling blankets. Watch for myoglobinuria.

2. Forty-five minutes after completion of a cystoscopy, a patient develops chills and a fever spike of 104° F.

This early on after an invasive procedure, and this high a fever, means bacteremia. Take blood cultures times 3, and start empiric antibiotic therapy.

3. On postoperative day 1 after an abdominal procedure, a patient develops a fever of 102°F.

Fever on day 1 means atelectasis, but all the other potential sources have to be ruled out. Management includes the following:

- Chest x-ray
- Look at wound and IV sites
- Inquire about urinary tract symptoms
- Improve ventilation: deep breathing and coughing, postural drainage, incentive spirometry

The ultimate therapy for major, recalcitrant atelectasis is bronchoscopy.

4. On postoperative day 1 after an abdominal procedure, a patient develops a fever of 102° F. The patient is not compliant with therapy for atelectasis, and by postoperative day 3 still has daily fever in the same range.

Now a pneumonic process has developed in the atelectatic segments. Chest x-ray, sputum cultures, and appropriate antibiotics are needed.

5. A patient who had major abdominal surgery is afebrile during the first 2 postoperative days, but on day 3 he has a fever spike to 103° F.

6. A patient who had major abdominal surgery is afebrile during the first 4 postoperative days, but on day 5 he has a fever spike to 103° F.

7. A patient who had major abdominal surgery is afebrile during the first 6 postoperative days, but on day 7 he has a fever spike to 103° F.

Every potential source of post-op fever always has to be investigated, but the timing of the first febrile episode gives a clue as to the most likely source. The mnemonic used (sequentially) is the "4 Ws": wind (for atelectasis), water (for urine), walking (for the veins in the leg), and wound. Thus UTI, thrombophlebitis, and wound infection are the likely culprits in these vignettes. Urinalysis and urinary culture, Doppler studies, and physical examination are the respective tests.

8. A patient who had major abdominal surgery has a normal postoperative course, with no significant episodes of fever, until the 10th day when his temperature begins to spike up to 102 and 103°F every day.

Now deep abscess (intra-abdominal: typically pelvic or subphrenic) is the most likely source, and CT scan is performed to diagnose; management is percutaneous drainage.

Chest Pain

9. On postoperative day 2 after an abdominoperineal resection for rectal cancer, a 72-year-old man complains of severe retrosternal pain, radiating to the left arm. He also becomes short of breath and tachycardic.

10. During the performance of an abdominoperineal resection for rectal cancer, unexpected severe bleeding is encountered, and the patient is hypotensive on and off for almost 1 hour. The anesthesiologist notes ST depression and T wave flattening in the ECG monitor.

Perioperative MI happens within the first 3 days, and the biggest triggering cause is hypovolemic shock. These two are fairly typical scenarios, although the classic chest pain picture is often obscured by other ongoing events. When thinking MI, everybody does an ECG, but the most reliable diagnostic test is serum troponin.

11. On postoperative day 7 after pinning of a broken hip, a 76-year-old man suddenly develops severe pleuritic chest pain and shortness of breath. When examined, he is found to be anxious, diaphoretic, and tachycardic, and he has prominent distended veins in his neck and forehead.

Chest pain this late post-op is pulmonary embolus (PE). This patient is obviously at high risk, and the findings are classic. If they give you a similar vignette in which the venous pressure is low, it virtually excludes this diagnosis. Arterial blood gases are your first test, and hypoxemia and hypocapnia are the obligatory findings (in their absence, it is not a PE either). CTA is the gold standard diagnostic test of choice. Therapy starts with heparinization. The very active natural fibrinolytic mechanism in the lung makes the use of clot-busters less clearly indicated, but if PEs recur during anticoagulation, a vena cava filter (Greenfield) is needed.

This man already had a PE. It is too late to think about preventive measures for him, but read the narrative portion of this book for a brief review of those.

Other Pulmonary Complications

12. An awake intubation is being attempted in a drunk and combative man who has sustained gunshot wounds to the abdomen. In the struggle the patient vomits and aspirates a large amount of gastric contents with particulate matter.

This is every anesthesiologist's nightmare. Aspiration can kill a patient right away, or produce chemical injury to the tracheobronchial tree ("chemical pneumonitis"). This is an inflammatory problem, not an infectious one, so antibiotics are not immediately indicated. However the irritation results in pulmonary failure and increases the risk of secondary pneumonia. Prevention is best (empty stomach, antacids before induction), but once it happens, lavage and removal of particulate matter is the first step (with the help of bronchoscopy), followed by bronchodilators and respiratory support. Steroids are not useful.

13. A trauma patient is undergoing a laparotomy for a seat belt injury. He also sustained several broken ribs. Halfway through the case it becomes progressively difficult to "bag" him, and his BP steadily declines, while the CVP steadily rises. There is no evidence of intraabdominal bleeding.

This patient has intraoperative tension pneumothorax. The lung was punctured by one of the broken ribs. The best approach is immediate thoracic needle decompression. The formal chest tube can be placed later.

Disorientation/Coma

14. Eighteen hours after major surgery, a patient becomes disoriented.

This is a very brief vignette, but out of the very long list of things that can produce post-op disorientation, the most lethal one if not promptly recognized and treated is hypoxia. So, unless it is clear from the vignette that we can blame metabolic problems (uremia, hyponatremia, hypernatremia, ammonium, hyperglycemia, delirium tremens [DTs], or our own medications), the safest thing to ask for first is blood gases.

15. In the second week of a stormy, complicated postoperative period in a young patient with multiple gunshot wounds to the abdomen, he becomes progressively disoriented and unresponsive. He has bilateral pulmonary infiltrates, and a PO_2 of 65 while breathing 40% oxygen. He has no evidence of CHF.

The reason for the mental changes are obvious: he is not getting enough oxygen in his blood, but the rest of the findings specifically identify adult respiratory distress syndrome (ARDS). The centerpiece of therapy for ARDS is PEEP, with care not to use too much volume, which may damage the lungs. Another issue is why does he have ARDS? In an older patient we can blame preexisting lung disease, and when there has been trauma to the chest, that can be the cause—but when those are not present, we have to think of sepsis as the precipitating event.

16. An alcoholic man checks in to have an elective colon resection for recurrent diverticular bleeding. He swears to everyone that he has not touched a drop of alcohol for the past 6 months. On postoperative day 3 he becomes disoriented and combative, and claims to see elephants crawling up the walls. The wife then reveals that the patient actually drank heavily up until the day of hospital admission.

These are obviously DTs. The standard management relies on benzodiazepines. In the past surgeons used IV alcohol (5% alcohol/5% dextrose), but this is most uncommon today. Most hospitals allow oral intake of alcohol for such scenarios.

17. Twelve hours after completion of an abdominal hysterectomy, a 42-year-old woman becomes confused and lethargic, complains of severe headache, has a grand mal seizure, and finally goes into a coma. Review of the chart reveals that an order for D5W, to run in at 125 ml/h, was mistakenly implemented as 525 ml/h.

This is a classic example of water intoxication. The laboratory finding that will confirm it will be a very low serum sodium concentration. Mortality for this iatrogenic condition is very high, and therapy is very controversial. Very careful use of hypertonic saline is probably a reasonable answer.

18. Eight hours after completion of a trans-sphenoidal hypophysectomy for a prolactinoma, a young woman becomes lethargic, confused, and eventually comatose. Review of the record shows that her urinary output since surgery has averaged 600 ml/h, although her IV fluids are going in at 100 ml/h.

The reverse of the previous vignette. Large, rapid, unreplaced water loss from surgically induced diabetes insipidus. The lab will show significant hypernatremia, and the safest therapy would use 1/3 or 1/4 normal saline to replace the lost fluid, although in this acute setting D5W would be acceptable.

19. A cirrhotic patient goes into coma after an emergency portocaval shunt for bleeding esophageal varices.

Brief but obvious: the culprit here will be ammonia. If there is also hypokalemic alkalosis and high cardiac output–low peripheral resistance, overt liver failure has occurred.

Urinary Complications

20. Six hours after undergoing a hemorrhoidectomy under spinal anesthesia, a 62-year-old man complains of suprapubic discomfort and fullness. He feels the need to void but has not been able to do so since the operation. There is a palpable suprapubic mass that is dull to percussion.

By far the most common post-op urinary problem is inability to void, and men are the likely victims. In-and-out bladder catheterization is the answer. Some authors recommend leaving an indwelling Foley catheter if catheterization has to be repeated in 6 hours, others wait until it has been done twice before suggesting it.

21. A man has had an abdominoperineal resection for cancer of the rectum, and an indwelling Foley catheter was left in place after surgery. The nurses are concerned because even though his vital signs have been stable, his urinary output in the last 2 hours has been zero.

In the presence of renal perfusing pressure, an output of zero invariably means a mechanical problem. In this case the catheter is plugged or kinked. More ominous—but much more rare—possibilities include both ureters having been tied off or thrombosis of the renal vessels.

22. Several hours after completion of multiple surgery for blunt trauma in an average-size adult, the urinary output is reported in 3 consecutive hours as 12 ml/h, 17 ml/h, and 9 ml/h. His BP has hovered around 95 to 130 systolic during that time.

His kidneys are perfusing, but he is either behind in fluid replacement or has gone into renal failure. A fluid challenge would suggest which situation exists. A bolus of 500 ml given in 10–20 minutes should produce diuresis in the dehydrated patient but not in renal failure.

The more elegant way, however, and the answer for the exam, is to look at urinary sodium. The dehydrated patient will be retaining sodium, and the urine will be <10 or 20 mEq/L. In renal failure the figure will be >40. An even more elegant calculation is the fractional excretion of sodium, which in renal failure >1.

Abdominal Distention

23. Four days after exploratory laparotomy for blunt abdominal trauma with resection and reanastomosis of damaged small bowel, a patient has abdominal distention, without abdominal pain. He has no bowel sounds and has not passed flatus, and his abdominal x-rays show dilated loops of small bowel without air fluid levels.

Probably paralytic ileus, which can be expected under the circumstances. NPO and NG suction should be continued until peristaltic activity resumes. Should resolution not be forthcoming, mechanical obstruction should be ruled out with a CT scan of the abdomen that will demonstrate a transition point between the proximal, dilated bowel and the distal collapsed bowel at the site of obstruction. Hypokalemia should also be ruled out.

24. An elderly gentleman with Alzheimer's disease who lived in a nursing home is operated on for a fractured femoral neck. On postoperative day 5 it is noted that his abdomen is grossly distended and tense, but not tender. He has occasional bowel sounds. X-rays show a very distended colon and a few distended loops of small bowel.

In the elderly who are not very active to begin with and are now further immobilized, massive colonic dilatation (Ogilvie syndrome) is commonly seen. Correct the fluids and electrolytes first. Neostigmine can dramatically improve colon motility, but it has significant side effects. Colonoscopy is a common successful treatment.

Wound

25. On postoperative day 5 after a laparotomy, it is noted that large amounts of salmon-colored clear fluid are soaking the dressings.

The classic presentation of a wound dehiscence. The patient must go to the OR for repair.

26. The nurses report that on postoperative day 5 after a laparotomy, a patient has been draining clear pink fluid from his abdominal wound. A medical student removes the dressing and asks the patient to sit up so he can get out of bed and be helped to the treatment room. When the patient complies, the wound opens widely and a handful of small bowel rushes out.

This one is evisceration, a rather serious problem. Put the patient back in bed, cover the bowel with large moist dressings soaked in warm saline (moist and warm are the key), and make arrangements to rush him to the OR for reclosure.

27. On postoperative day 7, the inguinal incision of an open inguinal herniorrhaphy is found to be red, hot, tender, and boggy (fluctuant). The patient reports fever for the past 2 days.

Wound infection. This far advanced there is sure to be pus, and the wound has to be opened. If it were just a bit of redness early on, antibiotics might still be able to abort the process. If there is doubt as to the presence or absence of pus, a sonogram is diagnostic.

28. Nine days after a sigmoid resection for cancer, the wound drains a brown fluid that everybody recognizes as feces. The patient is afebrile, and otherwise doing quite well.

A fecal fistula, if draining to the outside, is inconvenient but not serious. It will close eventually with little or no therapy. If feces were accumulating on the inside, the patient would be febrile and sick, and would need drainage and probably a diverting colostomy.

29. Eight days after a difficult hemigastrectomy and gastroduodenostomy for gastric ulcer, a patient begins to leak 2–3 L of green fluid per day through the right corner of his bilateral subcostal abdominal wound.

If patient is febrile, with an acute abdomen, and sick, he needs to be explored. The problem is serious. However, if all the gastric and duodenal contents are leaking to the outside, further immediate surgery is not the answer.

- Provide massive fluid and electrolyte replacement
- Provide nutritional support, with elemental nutrients delivered into the upper jejunum.
  - Total parenteral nutrition [TPN] is second choice but less effective and greater potential risk

The goal is eventual healing without having to operate again. The abdominal wall has to be protected from the digestion caused by the leaking GI fluids. Somatostatin or octreotide may diminish the volume of GI fluid loss.

Fluids and Electrolytes

30. Eight hours after completion of a trans-sphenoidal hypophysectomy for a prolactinoma, a young woman becomes lethargic, confused, and eventually comatose. Review of the record shows that her urinary output since surgery has averaged 600 ml/h, although her IV fluids are going in at 100 ml/h. A serum sodium determination shows a concentration of 152 mEq/L.

An elevated concentration of serum sodium invariably means that the patient has lost pure water (or hypotonic fluids). Every 3 mEq/L above the normal of 140 represents 1 L lost. This woman is 4 L shy, which fits her history of a diuresis of 500 ml/h more than the intake she is getting. As previously noted, she could be given 4 L of D5W, but many would prefer a similar amount of 5% dextrose in half normal saline, or 5% dextrose in one-third normal saline.

31. Several friends go on a weekend camping trip in the desert. On day 2 they lose their way as well as all connection via electronic devices. They are rescued a week later. One of them is brought to your hospital--awake and alert--with obvious clinical signs of dehydration. Serum sodium concentration is 155 mEq/L.

This gentleman has also lost water, about 5 L, but has done so slowly, by pulmonary and cutaneous evaporation over 5 days. He is hypernatremic, but his brain has adapted to the slowly changing situation. Were he to be given 5 L of D5W, the rapid correction of his hypertonicity would be dangerous. Five liters of 5% dextrose in half normal saline would be a much safer plan.

32. Twelve hours after completion of an abdominal hysterectomy, a 42-year-old woman becomes confused and lethargic, complains of severe headache, has a grand mal seizure, and finally goes into coma. Review of the chart reveals that an order for D5W to run in at 125 ml/h was mistakenly implemented as 525 ml/h. Her serum sodium concentration is 122 mEq/L.

In the surgical patient with normal kidneys, hyponatremia invariably means that water (without sodium) has been retained, thus the body fluids have been diluted. In this case a lot of IV water was given, and the antidiuretic hormone (ADH) produced as part of the metabolic response to trauma has held onto it. Rapidly developing hyponatremia (water intoxication) is a big problem (the brain has no time to adapt), and once it has occurred the therapy is very controversial. Most authors would recommend hypertonic saline (either 3% or 5%) given 100 ml at a time, and reassessing the situation (clinical and lab) before each succeeding dose.

33. A 62-year-old woman comes in for her scheduled chemotherapy administration for her metastatic cancer of the breast. Although she is quite asymptomatic, the lab reports that her serum sodium concentration is 122 mEq/L.

In this setting, water has also been retained (by ADH produced by the tumor), but so slowly that the brain has kept up with the developing hypotonicity. Rapid correction would be lethal and ill advised. Water restriction, on the other hand, will slowly allow the abnormality to be reversed.

34. A 68-year-old woman comes in with an obvious incarcerated umbilical hernia. She has gross abdominal distension, is clinically dehydrated, and reports persistent fecaloid vomiting for the past 5 days. She is awake and alert, and her serum sodium concentration is 118 mEq/L.

Hyponatremia means water retention, but in this case the problem began with loss of isotonic (sodium-containing) fluid from her gut. As her extracellular fluid became depleted, she has retained whatever water has come her way: tea and Coke that she still was able to drink early on, and endogenous water from catabolism. Thus she is now volume-depleted at the same time that she is hyponatremic (hypotonic). She desperately needs volume replacement, but we do not want to correct her hypotonicity too quickly. Thus lots of isotonic fluids (start with 1 or 2 L/h of normal saline or Ringer's lactate, depending on her acid-base status) would be the way to go (use clinical variables to fine-tune). Once her volume is replenished, she will unload the retained water and correct her own tonicity.

35. A patient with severe diabetic ketoacidosis comes in with profound dehydration and a serum potassium concentration 5.2 mEq/L. After several hours of vigorous therapy with insulin and IV fluids (saline, without potassium), his serum potassium concentration is reported as 2.9.

Severe acidosis (or alkalosis, for that matter) results in the loss of potassium in the urine. While the acidosis is present, though, the serum concentration is high because potassium has come out of the cells in exchange for hydrogen ion. Once the acidosis is corrected, that potassium rushes back into the cells, and the true magnitude of the potassium loss becomes evident. He obviously needs potassium. (Under most circumstances, 10 mEq/h is a safe "speed limit." In this setting, 20 mEq/h can be justified.)

36. An 18-year-old woman slips and falls under a bus, and her right leg is crushed. On arrival at the ED she is hypotensive, and she receives several units of blood. Over the next several hours she is in and out of hypovolemic shock, and she develops acidosis. Her serum potassium concentration, which was 4.8 mEq/L at the time of admission, is reported to be 6.1 a few hours later.

Let's count the ways in which potassium has been pouring into her blood: it came out of the crushed leg, it came in with the blood transfusions, and it came from the cells when she became acidotic. With low perfusing pressure (in and out of shock), the kidneys have not been doing a great job of eliminating it. We will have to do that. In addition to improving her BP, we can "push potassium into the cells" with insulin and 50% dextrose. We can help dispose of it with exchange resins, and we can neutralize it with IV calcium. Hemodialysis is the ultimate weapon.

37. An elderly alcoholic, diabetic man, with marginal renal function, sustains multiple trauma while driving under the influence of alcohol. In the course of his resuscitation and multiple surgeries, he is in and out of shock for prolonged periods of time. Blood gases show a pH of 7.1 and Pco2 of 36. His serum electrolytes are sodium 138, chloride 98, and bicarbonate 15.

This man has every reason to develop metabolic acidosis, and he will do so by retention of fixed acids (rather than by loss of bicarbonate). The main driving force in this case is the state of shock, with lactic acid production; but the diabetes, alcohol, and bad kidney are also contributing.

The lab shows that indeed he has metabolic acidosis (low pH and low bicarbonate), he is trying to compensate by hyperventilating (low Pco2), and he shows the classic anion gap (the sum of his chloride and bicarbonate is 25 mEq shy of the serum sodium concentration—instead of the normal 10 to 15).

As for the therapy, the classic treatment for metabolic acidosis is either bicarbonate or a bicarbonate precursor such as lactate or acetate. But in cases like this, reliance on such therapy tends to eventually produce alkalosis once the low flow state is corrected. Thus the emphasis here should be in fluid resuscitation. However, the choice of fluid is critical: a lot of saline would not be a good idea (too much chloride). A lot of Ringer's lactate would be a better choice.

38. A patient who has had a subtotal gastrectomy for cancer, with a Billroth 2 reconstruction, develops a "blowout" of the duodenal stump, and a subsequent duodenal fistula. For the past 10 days he has been draining 750–1,500 mL/d of green fluid. His serum electrolytes show sodium 132, chloride 104, and bicarbonate 15. The pH in his blood is 7.2, with Pco_2 35.

Again, metabolic acidosis, but now with a normal anion gap. He has been losing lots of bicarbonate out of the fistula. The problem would not have developed if his IV fluid replacement had contained lots of bicarbonate (or lactate, or acetate), but the use of those agents is indicated now for the therapy of the existing abnormality.

39. A patient with severe peptic ulcer disease develops pyloric obstruction and has protracted vomiting of clear gastric contents (i.e., without bile) for several days. His serum electrolytes show sodium 134, chloride 82, potassium 2.9, and bicarbonate 34.

The classic hypochloremic, hypokalemic, metabolic alkalosis secondary to loss of acid gastric juice. This man needs to be rehydrated (choose saline rather than Ringer's lactate), and he needs lots of potassium chloride (10 mEq/h will give him plenty, and will be a safe rate). Very rarely is ammonium chloride (or diluted, buffered hydrochloric acid) needed.

General Surgery 4

DISEASES OF THE GASTROINTESTINAL SYSTEM

Upper Gastrointestinal System

Esophagus

1. A 62-year-old man describes epigastric and substernal pain that he cannot characterize well. At times his description sounds like gastroesophageal reflux, at times it does not. Sonogram of the gallbladder, ECG, and cardiac enzymes have been negative.

What is it? The question is, is it gastroesophageal reflux?

Diagnosis. Esophageal pH monitoring.

2. A 54-year-old obese man gives a history of burning retrosternal pain and heartburn that is brought about by bending over, wearing tight clothing, or lying flat in bed at night. He gets symptomatic relief from antacids but has never been formally treated. The problem has been present for many years, and seems to be progressing.

What is it? The description is classic for gastroesophageal reflux disease (GERD).

Management. The diagnosis is not really in doubt, and with that clinical picture alone thousands of patients are treated with symptomatic medication—but the academicians writing exam questions would want you to recommend endoscopy and biopsies to assess the extent of esophagitis and potential complications, specifically, Barrett's esophagus.

3. A 54-year-old obese man gives a history of burning retrosternal pain and heartburn that is brought about by bending over, wearing tight clothing, or lying flat in bed at night. He gets symptomatic relief from antacids but has never been formally treated. The problem has been present for many years, and seems to be progressing. Endoscopy shows severe peptic esophagitis and Barrett's esophagus.

Management for Barrett's has evolved, and the diagnosis alone is no longer considered an indication for surgery. In this patient who has not had formal medical management, that should be the first step. Continued symptoms would warrant consideration for fundoplication. Dysplastic changes would require resection.

4. A 54-year-old obese man gives a history of many years of burning retrosternal pain and heartburn that is brought about by bending over, wearing tight clothing, or lying flat in bed at night. He gets brief symptomatic relief from antacids, but in spite of faithful adherence to a strict program of medical therapy, the process seems to be progressing. Endoscopy shows severe peptic esophagitis with no dysplastic changes.

Management: He has failed medical management, and has no dysplastic changes. He needs a fundoplication. Whether or not it is performed, he needs endoscopy surveillance with biopsies to follow progression of the esophagitis.

5. A 47-year-old woman describes difficulty swallowing, which she has had for many years. She says that liquids are more difficult to swallow than solids, and she has learned to sit up straight and wait for the fluids to "make it through." Occasionally she regurgitates large amounts of undigested food.

It sure sounds like achalasia. The diagnosis is suggested by a barium swallow (usually the first test) and confirmed by manometry studies. Endoscopic Botox injection, balloon dilation and surgery are the therapeutic options.

6. A 54-year-old black man with a history of smoking and drinking describes progressive dysphagia that began 3 months ago with difficulty swallowing meat, progressed to other solid foods, then soft foods, and is now evident for liquids as well. He locates the place where the food "sticks" at the lower end of the sternum. He has lost 30 pounds of weight.

A classic for carcinoma of the esophagus (progressive dysphagia, weight loss). Given the detail of race, age, sex, and habits, it is probably squamous cell cancer. Had the history been long-standing reflux, it would suggest adenocarcinoma.

The diagnosis is made the same way for both: endoscopy and biopsies—but the endoscopist wants a "road map" first. The sequence is barium swallow, then endoscopy with U/S and biopsies, then CT scan (to assess extent and limitations to respectability such as metastatic disease).

7. A 24-year-old man spends the night cruising bars and drinking heavily. In the wee hours of the morning he is quite drunk, and he starts vomiting repeatedly. He initially brings up gastric contents only, but eventually he vomits bright red blood.

8. A 24-year-old man spends the night cruising bars and drinking heavily. In the wee hours of the morning he is quite drunk and starts vomiting repeatedly. Eventually he has a particularly violent episode of vomiting, and he feels a very severe, wrenching epigastric pain and low sternal pain of sudden onset. On arrival at the ED 1 hour later he still has the pain, is diaphoretic, has fever and leukocytosis, and looks quite ill.

What is it? Two vignettes that have the same beginnings, with one leading to bleeding (Mallory-Weiss tear), and the other one to perforation (Boerhaave syndrome).

Management. For the patient who is bleeding, endoscopy to ascertain the diagnosis and occasionally treat. Bleeding will typically be arterial and brisk, but self-limiting. Photocoagulation can be used if needed, and rarely a discrect mucosal tear is identified that can be clipped. The patient with perforation is facing a potentially lethal problem. Gastrografin swallow will confirm the diagnosis, and emergency surgical repair will follow. Prognosis depends on time elapsed between perforation and treatment, and degree of mediastinal contamination that has occurred.

9. A 66-year-old man has an upper GI endoscopy done as an outpatient to check on the progress of medical therapy for gastric ulcer. Six hours after the procedure, he returns complaining of severe, constant retrosternal pain that began shortly after he went home. He looks prostrate and very ill, is diaphoretic, has a fever of 104°F, and a respiratory rate of 30. There is a hint of subcutaneous emphysema at the base of the neck.

What is it? Instrumental perforation of the esophagus. The setting plus the air in the tissues are virtually diagnostic. Do Gastrografin swallow and emergency surgical repair. Severe pain after endoscopy is a perforation until proven otherwise.

Stomach

10. A 72-year-old man has lost 40 pounds of weight over a 2- or 3-month period. He gives a history of anorexia for several months, and of vague epigastric discomfort for the past 3 weeks.

What is it? Cancer of the stomach is a possibility, along with other etiologies.

Diagnosis. Imaging studies followed by endoscopy and biopsies.

Management. Surgery will be done for cure if possible, for palliation if not.

Mid and Lower Gastrointestinal System

Small bowel and appendix

11. A 54-year-old man has had colicky abdominal pain and protracted vomiting for several days. He has developed progressive moderate abdominal distention, and has not had a bowel movement or passed any gas for 5 days. He has high-pitched, loud bowel sounds that coincide with the colicky pain, and x-rays show distended loops of small bowel and air-fluid levels. Five years ago he had an exploratory laparotomy for a gunshot wound of the abdomen.

What is it? Mechanical intestinal obstruction, caused by adhesions.

Management. NG suction, IV fluids, and careful observation.

12. A 54-year-old man has had colicky abdominal pain and protracted vomiting for several days. He has developed progressive moderate abdominal distention, and has not had a bowel movement or passed any gas for 5 days. He has high-pitched, loud bowel sounds that coincide with the colicky pain, and x-rays show distended loops of small bowel and air-fluid levels. Five years ago he had an exploratory laparotomy for a gunshot wound of the abdomen. Six hours after being hospitalized and placed on NG suction and IV fluids, he develops fever, leukocytosis, abdominal tenderness, and rebound tenderness.

What is it? He has strangulated obstruction, i.e., a loop of bowel is dying—or dead—from compression of the mesenteric blood supply.

Management. Emergency surgery.

13. A 54-year-old man has had colicky abdominal pain and protracted vomiting for several days. He has developed progressive moderate abdominal distention, and has not had a bowel movement or passed any gas for 5 days. He has high-pitched, loud bowel sounds that coincide with the colicky pain, and x-rays show distended loops of small bowel and air-fluid levels. On physical examination a groin mass is noted, and he explains that he used to be able to "push it back" at will, but for the past 5 days has been unable to do so.

What is it? Mechanical intestinal obstruction caused by an incarcerated (potentially strangulated) hernia.

Management. After suitable fluid replacement he needs urgent surgical intervention.

14. A 55-year-old woman is being evaluated for protracted diarrhea. On further questioning she gives a bizarre history of episodes of flushing of the face, with expiratory wheezing. A prominent jugular venous pulse is noted on her neck.

What is it? Carcinoid syndrome.

Diagnosis. Twenty-four-hour urinary collection for 5-hydroxy-indolacetic acid, perform a CT scan to assess liver metastasis, and plan resection based upon the results.

15. A 22-year-old man develops anorexia followed by vague periumbilical pain that several hours later becomes sharp, severe, constant, and well localized to the right lower quadrant of the abdomen. He has abdominal tenderness, guarding, and rebound to the right and below the umbilicus, temperature 99.6° F, and white blood cell count 12,500, with neutrophilia and immature forms.

What is it? A classic for acute appendicitis.

Management. Perform emergency appendectomy. If the case had not been typical, do CT scan. In children and women of child-bearing age for whom the presentation is not typical, U/S can also make the diagnosis and prevent radiation exposure,

Colon

16. A 59-year-old man is referred for evaluation because he has been fainting at his job where he operates heavy machinery. He is pale and gaunt, but otherwise his physical examination is remarkable only for 4+ occult blood in the stool. Lab shows hemoglobin 5 g/dl.

What is it? Cancer of the right colon.

Diagnosis. Colonoscopy and biopsies.

Management. Blood transfusions and eventually right hemicolectomy.

17. A 56-year-old man has bloody bowel movements. The blood coats the outside of the stool, and has been present on and off for several weeks. For the past 2 months he has been constipated, and his stools have become of narrow caliber.

What is it? Cancer of the distal, left side of the colon.

Diagnosis. Endoscopy and biopsies. If given choices, start with flexible proctosigmoidoscopy (with the 45-cm or 60-cm instrument that any MD can handle). Eventually full colonoscopy (to rule out a second primary) will be needed before surgery.

18. A 77-year-old man has a colonoscopy because of rectal bleeding. A villous adenoma is found in the rectum, and several adenomatous polyps are identified in the sigmoid and descending colon.

The issue with polyps is which ones are premalignant, and thus need to be excised. Premalignant include, in descending order of potential for malignant conversion, familial polyposis (and all variants, such as Gardner), familial multiple inflammatory polyps, villous adenoma, and adenomatous polyp. Benign polyps, which can be left alone, include juvenile, Peutz-Jeghers, isolated, inflammatory, and hyperplastic.

19. A 42-year-old man has suffered from chronic ulcerative colitis for 20 years. He weighs 90 pounds and has had at least 40 hospital admissions for exacerbations of the disease. Because of a recent relapse, he has been placed on high-dose steroids and Imuran. For the past 12 hours he has had severe abdominal pain, temperature of 104°F, and leukocytosis. He looks ill and "toxic." His abdomen is tender, particularly in the epigastric area, and he has muscle guarding and rebound. X-rays show a massively distended transverse colon, and there is gas within the wall of the colon.

What is it? Toxic megacolon.

Management. Emergency surgery for the toxic megacolon, but the case illustrates all of the other indications for surgery in chronic ulcerative colitis. The involved colon has to be removed, and that always includes the rectal mucosa.

20. A 27-year-old man is recovering from an appendectomy for gangrenous acute appendicitis with perforation and periappendicular abscess. He has been receiving Clindamycin and Tobramycin for 7 days. Eight hours ago he developed watery diarrhea, crampy abdominal pain, fever, and leukocytosis.

What is it? Pseudomembranous colitis from overgrowth of *Clostridium difficile*.

Diagnosis. The diagnosis relies primarily on identification of toxin in the stools. Cultures take too long, and proctosigmoidoscopic exam does not always find typical changes.

Management. Clindamycin has to be stopped, and antidiarrheal medications (diphenoxylate combined with atropine, paregoric) should not be used. Metronidazole is the usual drug of choice. An alternate drug is vancomycin. Failure of medical management, with a marked leukocytosis and serum lactate above 5 mmol/L, is an indication for emergency colectomy.

Anorectal Disease

21. A 60-year-old man known to have hemorrhoids reports bright red blood on the toilet paper after evacuation.

22. A 60-year-old man known to have hemorrhoids complains of anal itching and discomfort, particularly toward the end of the day. He has mild perianal pain when sitting down and finds himself sitting sideways to avoid the discomfort.

What is it? The rule is that internal hemorrhoids bleed but do not hurt, whereas external hemorrhoids hurt but do not bleed.

Management. It is not reassurance and hemorrhoid remedies prescribed over the phone! In all anorectal problems, cancer has to be ruled out first. The correct answer is proctosigmoidoscopic examination (digital rectal exam, anoscopy, and flexible sigmoidoscope). Once the diagnosis has been confirmed, internal hemorrhoids can be treated with rubber-band ligation, whereas external hemorrhoids or prolapsed hemorrhoids require surgery.

23. A 23-year-old woman describes exquisite pain with defecation and blood streaks on the outside of the stools. Because of the pain she avoids having bowel movements and when she finally does, the stools are hard and even more painful. Physical examination cannot be done, as she refuses to allow anyone to even draw apart her buttocks to look at the anus for fear of precipitating the pain.

A classic description of anal fissure. Even though the clinical picture is classic, cancer still has to be ruled out. Examination under anesthesia is the correct answer. Medical management includes stool softeners and topical agents. A tight sphincter is believed to cause and perpetuate the problem, and injections with paralyzing agents (botulin toxin) have been proposed. If it gets to surgery, lateral internal sphincterotomy is the operation of choice.

Fissures are preferably treated by calcium channel blockers such as diltiazem ointment 2% topically 3x/daily for 6 weeks, or cortisone suppositories. They have an 80-90% success rate. Botox has a 50% rate of healing.

24. A 28-year-old man is brought to the office by his mother. In the last 4 months he has had 3 operations—done elsewhere—for a perianal fistula, though after each one the area has not healed, and in fact the surgical wounds have become bigger. The patient now has multiple unhealing ulcers, fissures, and fistulas all around the anus, with purulent discharge. There are no palpable masses.

Another classic. The perianal area has a fantastic blood supply and heals beautifully even though feces bathe the wounds. When it does not, immediately think of Crohn's disease.

You must still rule out malignancy (anal cancer does not heal either if not completely excised). A proper examination with biopsies is needed. The specimens should confirm Crohn's. Fistulotomy is not recommended. Most fistulae will get draining setons which will ensure adequate drainage of infection while medical management controls the disease. Remicade in particular has shown to help heal these fistulae.

25. A 44-year-old man shows up in the ED at 11 pm with exquisite perianal pain. He cannot sit down, reports that bowel movements are very painful, and has been having chills and fever. Physical examination shows a hot, tender, red, fluctuant mass between the anus and the ischial tuberosity.

Another very common problem: ischiorectal abscess. The treatment for all abscesses is drainage. This one is no exception. But cancer also has to be ruled out. Thus the best option would be an answer that offers examination under anesthesia and incision and drainage. If the patient is diabetic, incision and drainage would have to be followed by very close in-hospital follow-up.

26. A 62-year-old man complains of perianal discomfort and reports that there are fecal streaks soiling his underwear. Four months ago he had a perirectal abscess drained surgically. Physical examination shows a perianal opening in the skin, and a cordlike tract can be palpated going from the opening toward the inside of the anal canal. Brownish purulent discharge can be expressed from the tract.

What is it? A pretty good description of fistula-in-ano.

Management. First rule out cancer with proctosigmoidoscopy (necrotic tumors can drain). Then schedule elective fistulotomy.

27. A 55-year-old HIV-positive man has a fungating mass growing out of the anus, and rock-hard, enlarged lymph nodes in both groins. He has lost a lot of weight, and looks emaciated and ill.

What is it? Squamous cell carcinoma of the anus.

Diagnosis. Biopsies of the fungating mass.

Management. Nigro protocol is combined preoperative chemotherapy and radiation for 5 weeks with 90% cure rate. Surgery is done only if Nigro fails to cure the cancer.

Gastrointestinal Bleeding

28. A 33-year-old man vomits a large amount of bright red blood.

What is it? Pretty skimpy vignette, but you can already define the territory where the bleeding is taking place: from the tip of the nose to the ligament of Treitz.

Diagnosis. Don't forget to look at the mouth and nose and then proceed with upper GI endoscopy.

29. A 33-year-old man has had 3 large bowel movements that he describes as made up entirely of dark red blood. The last one was 20 minutes ago. He is diaphoretic and pale, and has a BP of 90 over 70 and pulse rate of 110.

The point of the vignette is that something needs to be done to define the area from which he is bleeding: with the available information, it could be from anywhere in the GI tract (a vast territory to investigate). Fortunately, he seems to be bleeding right now, thus the first diagnostic move is to place an NG tube and aspirate after you have looked at the nose and mouth.

30. A 33-year-old man has had 3 large bowel movements that he describes as made up entirely of dark red blood. The last one was 20 minutes ago. He is diaphoretic and pale, and has a BP of 90 over 70 and a pulse rate of 110. An NG tube returns copious amounts of bright red blood.

What is it? The area has been defined (tip of the nose to ligament of Treitz). Proceed with endoscopy.

31. A 65-year-old man has had 3 large bowel movements that he describes as made up entirely of dark red blood. The last one was 20 minutes ago. He is diaphoretic and pale, and has a BP of 90 over 70 and a pulse rate of 110. An NG tube returns clear, green fluid without blood.

What is it? If the NG tube had returned blood, the boundaries would have been tip of the nose to ligament of Treitz. Clear fluid, without bile, would have exonerated the area down to the pylorus, and if there is bile in the aspirate, down to the ligament of Treitz—provided you are sure that the patient is bleeding now. That's the case here. So, he is bleeding from somewhere distal to the ligament of Treitz.

Further definition of the actual site is no longer within reach of upper endoscopy, and except for anoscopy looking for bleeding hemorrhoids, lower endoscopy is notoriously unrewarding during massive bleeding. If he is bleeding at >2 ml/min (about 1 U of blood every 4 hours), some physicians go straight to the emergency angiogram. Those same physicians would wait and do a colonoscopy later if the bleeding is <0.5 mL/min, and they would resort to a tagged red-cell study for the cases in between. There is another school of thought that always begins with the tagged red-cell study, regardless of estimated rate of bleeding. If the question offers that choice in this setting (upper GI source has been ruled out, and bleeding hemorrhoids have been sought), it would be safe to pick it.

32. A 72-year-old man had 3 large bowel movements that he describes as made up entirely of dark red blood. The last one was 2 days ago. He is pale, but has normal vital signs. An NG tube returns clear, green fluid without blood.

What is it? The clear aspirate is meaningless because he is not bleeding right now. So the guilty territory can be anywhere from the tip of the nose to the anal canal. Across the board, 75% of all GI bleeding is upper, and virtually all the causes of lower GI bleeding are diseases of the old: diverticulosis, polyps, cancer, and angiodysplasias. So, when the patient is young, the odds overwhelmingly favor an upper site. When the patient is old, the overall preponderance of upper is balanced by the concentration of lower causes in old people—so it could be anywhere.

Diagnosis. Angiography is not the first choice for slow bleeding or bleeding that has stopped. Even the proponents of radionuclide studies don't have much hope if the patient bled 3 days ago. The first choice now is endoscopies, both upper and lower.

33. A 7-year-old boy passes a large bloody bowel movement.

What is it? In this age group, Meckel diverticulum leads the list.

Diagnosis. By radioactively labeled technetium scan (not the one that tags red cells, but the one that identifies gastric mucosa).

34. A 41-year-old man has been in the ICU for 2 weeks being treated for idiopathic hemorrhagic pancreatitis. He has had several percutaneous drainage procedures for pancreatic abscesses, chest tubes for pleural effusions, and bronchoscopies for atelectasis. He has been in and out of septic shock and respiratory failure several times. Ten minutes ago he vomited a large amount of bright red blood, and as you approach him he vomits again what looks like another pint of blood.

What is it? In this setting it has to be stress ulcer.

Management. It should have been prevented by keeping the pH of the stomach above 4 with H2 blockers, antacids, or both; but once the bleeding takes place, the diagnosis is made as usual with endoscopy. Treatment will be difficult (start with endoscopic attempts—laser and such), and it may require angiographic embolization of the left gastric artery.

Acute Abdomen

35. A 59-year-old man arrives in the ED at 2 AM, accompanied by his wife who is wearing curlers on her hair and a robe over her nightgown. He has abdominal pain that began suddenly about 1 hour ago, and is now generalized, constant, and extremely severe. He lies motionless on the stretcher, is diaphoretic, and has shallow, rapid breathing. His abdomen is rigid, very tender to deep palpation, and has guarding and rebound tenderness in all quadrants.

What is it? Definitely an acute abdomen. The time and circumstances attest to the severity and rapid onset of the problem. The physical findings are impressive. He has generalized acute peritonitis. The best bet is perforated peptic ulcer—but we do not need to prove that.

Management. The acute abdomen does not need a precise diagnosis to proceed with surgical exploration. Lower lobe pneumonia and MI have to be ruled out with chest x-ray and ECG, and it would be nice to have a plain x-ray or CT scan of the abdomen and a normal lipase—but the best answer of this vignette should be prompt emergency exploratory laparotomy.

36. A 62-year-old man with cirrhosis of the liver and ascites presents with generalized abdominal pain that started 12 hours ago. He now has moderate tenderness over the entire abdomen, with some guarding and equivocal rebound. He has mild fever and leukocytosis.

What is it? Peritonitis in the cirrhotic with ascites, or the child with nephrosis and ascites, could be spontaneous bacterial peritonitis—which does not need surgery—rather than acute peritonitis secondary to an intraabdominal catastrophe that requires emergency operation. This is very uncommon.

Diagnosis. Cultures of the ascitic fluid (aspirate via paracentesis) will yield a single organism. Treatment will be with the appropriate antibiotics.

37. A 43-year-old man develops excruciating abdominal pain at 8:18 PM. When seen in the ED at 8:50 PM, he has a rigid abdomen, lies motionless on the examining table, has no bowel sounds, and is obviously in great pain, which he describes as constant. X-ray shows free air under the diaphragm.

What is it? Acute abdomen plus perforated viscus equals perforated duodenal ulcer in most cases. Although I am exaggerating the sudden onset by giving the exact minute, vignettes of perforated peptic ulcer will have a pretty sharp time of onset.

Management. Emergency exploratory laparotomy.

38. A 44-year-old alcoholic man presents with severe epigastric pain that began shortly after a heavy bout of alcoholic intake, and reached maximum intensity over a period of 2 hours. The pain is constant, radiates straight through to the back, and is accompanied by nausea, vomiting, and retching.

He had a similar episode 2 years ago, for which he required hospitalization.

What is it? Acute pancreatitis.

Diagnosis. Serum amylase and lipase determinations. CT scan will follow if the diagnosis is unclear, or in a day or two if there is no improvement.

Management. NPO, NG suction, IV fluids.

39. A 43-year-old obese mother of 6 children has severe right upper quadrant abdominal pain that began 6 hours ago. The pain was colicky at first, radiated to the right shoulder and around toward the back, and was accompanied by nausea and vomiting. For the past 2 hours the pain has been constant. She has tenderness to deep palpation, muscle guarding, and rebound in the right upper quadrant. Her temperature is 101°F, and she has a WBC count of 16,000. She has had similar episodes of pain in the past brought about by ingestion of fatty food, but they all had been of brief duration and relented spontaneously or with anticholinergic medications.

What is it? Acute cholecystitis.

Diagnosis. Sonogram should be the first choice. If equivocal, an HIDA scan (radionuclide excretion scan) should be done.

Management. Start medical management (antibiotics, NPO, IV fluids) with the intention of doing laparoscopic cholecystectomy within the same hospital admission.

40. A 52-year-old man has right flank colicky pain of sudden onset that radiates to the inner thigh and scrotum. There is microscopic hematuria.

What is it? Ureteral colic (included here for differential diagnosis).

Diagnosis. Specific CT scan for ureteric colic is CT-KUB. This is a noncontrast CT scan that allows for visualization of a ureteric calculus.

41. A 59-year-old woman has a history of 3 prior episodes of left lower quadrant abdominal pain for which she was briefly hospitalized and treated with antibiotics. She began to feel discomfort 12 hours ago, and now she has constant left lower quadrant pain, tenderness, and a vaguely palpable mass.

    She has fever and leukocytosis.

What is it? Acute diverticulitis.

Diagnosis. In acute diverticulitis, CT scan is the gold standard investigation. After 6 weeks of cooling off, however, all cases must get a colonoscopy to rule out perforated colon cancer.

Management. Treatment is medical for the acute attack (antibiotics, NPO), but elective sigmoid resection is advisable for recurrent disease (like this woman is having). Percutaneous drainage of abscess is indicated if one is present. Emergency surgery (resection or colostomy) may be needed if she gets worse or does not respond to treatment.

42. An 82-year-old man develops severe abdominal distension, nausea, vomiting, and colicky abdominal pain. He has not passed any gas or stool for the past 12 hours. He has a tympanitic abdomen with hyperactive bowel sounds. X-ray shows distended loops of small and large bowel, and a very large gas shadow that is located in the right upper quadrant and tapers toward the left lower quadrant with the shape of a parrot's beak.

What is it? Volvulus of the sigmoid.

Management. Endoscopic intervention will relieve the obstruction. Eventually, surgery to prevent recurrences should be considered. If the patient has an acute abdomen, this means dead gut, and laparotomy is mandated.

43. A 79-year-old man with atrial fibrillation develops an acute abdomen. He has a silent abdomen, with diffuse tenderness and mild rebound. There is a trace of blood in the rectal exam. He has acidosis and looks quite sick. X-rays show distended small bowel and distended colon up to the middle of the transverse colon.

What is it? Acute abdomen in an elderly person who has atrial fibrillation brings to mind embolic occlusion of the mesenteric vessels. Acidosis frequently ensues, and blood in the stool is often seen. Unfortunately not much can be done, as the bowel is usually dead. Young, aggressive vascular surgeons would call for an angiogram to perform emergency embolectomy, assuming the case is seen very early before the bowel dies.

Hepatobiliary

Liver

44. A 53-year-old man with cirrhosis of the liver develops malaise, vague right upper quadrant abdominal discomfort, and 20-pound weight loss. Physical examination shows a palpable mass that seems to arise from the left lobe of the liver. α-fetoprotein is significantly elevated.

45. A 53-year-old man develops vague right upper quadrant abdominal discomfort and a 20-pound weight loss. Physical examination shows a palpable liver with nodularity. Two years ago he had a right hemicolectomy for cancer of the ascending colon. His carcinoembryonic antigen (CEA) had been within normal limits right after his hemicolectomy, but is now 10 times normal.

What is it? Both are good descriptions of cancer in the liver, included to remind you that α-fetoprotein goes with primary hepatoma, whereas CEA goes with metastatic tumor from the colon.

Diagnosis. Both would start with CT scan (with contrast) to define location and extent of tumor.

Management. In the primary hepatoma, resection would be performed if a tumor-free anatomic segment can be left behind. In the metastatic tumor, resection is done if there are no other metastases, it is surgically possible, and the primary is relatively slow growing.

46. A 24-year-old woman develops moderate, generalized abdominal pain of sudden onset, and shortly thereafter faints. At the time of evaluation in the ED she is pale, tachycardic, and hypotensive. The abdomen is mildly distended and tender, and she has hemoglobin 7 g/dl. There is no history of trauma. On inquiring as to whether she might be pregnant, she denies the possibility because she has been on birth control pills since she was age 14, and has never missed taking them.

What is it? Bleeding from a ruptured hepatic adenoma, secondary to birth control pills.

Management. It's pretty clear that she is bleeding into the belly, but CT scan will confirm it and probably show the liver adenoma as well. Surgery will follow. She will not be allowed to take birth control pills in the future.

47. A 44-year-old woman is recovering from an episode of acute ascending cholangitis secondary to choledocholithiasis. She develops fever and leukocytosis and some tenderness in the right upper quadrant. A sonogram reveals a liver abscess.

Not much of a diagnostic challenge here, but the issue is management, and it is included to contrast it with the handling of the patient in the next vignette. This is a pyogenic abscess, it needs to be drained which can usually be done by the radiologists percutaneously, other laparoscopic drainage can be performed.

48. A 29-year-old migrant worker from Mexico develops fever and leukocytosis, as well as tenderness over the liver when the area is percussed. He has mild jaundice and an elevated alkaline phosphatase. Sonogram of the right upper abdominal area shows a normal biliary tree and an abscess in the liver.

What is it? This one is an amebic abscess—very common in Mexico.

Management. Alone among abscesses, this one in most cases does not have to be drained, but can be effectively treated with Metronidazole. Get serology for amebic titers, but don't wait for the report (it will take 3 weeks). Start the patient on Metronidazole. Prompt improvement will tell you that you are on the right track. When the serologies come back, the patient will be well and your diagnosis will be confirmed. Don't fall for an option that suggests aspirating the pus and sending it for culture; you cannot grow the ameba from the pus.

Jaundice

49. A 42-year-old woman is jaundiced. She has a total bilirubin of 6, and laboratory reports that the unconjugated, indirect bilirubin is 6 and the direct, conjugated bilirubin is 0. She has no bile in the urine.

What is it? The vignette in the exam will be adorned with other evidence of hemolysis, but you do not need it to make the diagnosis. This is hemolytic jaundice.

Management. Try to figure out what is chewing her red cells.

50. A 19-year-old college student returns from a trip to Cancun, and 2 weeks later develops malaise, weakness, and anorexia. A week later he notices jaundice.

When he presents for evaluation his total bilirubin is 12, with 7 indirect and 5 direct. His alkaline phosphatase is mildly elevated, and the transaminases are very high.

What is it? Hepatocellular jaundice.

Management. Get serologies to confirm diagnosis and type of hepatitis.

51. A patient with progressive jaundice that has been present for 4 weeks is found to have a total bilirubin of 22, with 16 direct and 6 indirect, and minimally elevated transaminases. The alkaline phosphatase was twice the normal value 2 weeks ago, and now is about 6 times the upper limit of normal.

What is it? A generic example of obstructive jaundice.

Management. Sonogram, looking for dilated intrahepatic ducts, possibly dilated extrahepatic ducts as well, and if we get lucky, a finding of gallstones.

52. A 40-year-old obese mother of 5 children presents with progressive jaundice, which she first noticed 4 weeks ago. She has a total bilirubin of 22, with 16 direct and 6 indirect, and minimally elevated transaminases. The alkaline phosphatase is about 6 times the upper limit of normal. She gives a history of multiple episodes of colicky right upper quadrant abdominal pain, brought about by ingestion of fatty food.

What is it? Again, obstructive jaundice, with a good chance of being caused by stones.

Management. Start with the sonogram. If you need more tests after that, endoscopic retrograde cholangiopancreatography (ERCP) is the next move, which could also be used to remove the stones from the common duct. Cholecystectomy will eventually have to be performed.

53. A 66-year-old man presents with progressive jaundice, which he first noticed 6 weeks ago. He has total bilirubin of 22, with 16 direct and 6 indirect, and minimally elevated transaminases. The alkaline phosphatase is about 6 times the upper limit of normal. He has lost 10 pounds over the past 2 months, but is otherwise asymptomatic. A sonogram shows dilated intrahepatic ducts, dilated extrahepatic ducts, and a very distended, thin-walled gallbladder.

What is it? Malignant obstructive jaundice. "Silent" obstructive jaundice is more likely to be caused by tumor (although most patients with pancreatic tumor have dull constant pain). A distended gallbladder is an ominous sign: when stones are the source of the problem, the gallbladder is thick-walled and nonpliable.

Diagnosis. You already have the sonogram. Next move is CT scan. Follow with ERCP if the CT is not diagnostic.

54. A 66-year-old man presents with progressive jaundice, which he first noticed 6 weeks ago. He has a total bilirubin of 22, with 16 direct and 6 indirect, and minimally elevated transaminases. The alkaline phosphatase is about 6 times the upper limit of normal. He is otherwise asymptomatic. A sonogram shows dilated intrahepatic ducts, dilated extrahepatic ducts, and a very distended, thin-walled gallbladder. Except for the dilated ducts, the CT scan is unremarkable. ERCP shows a narrow area in the distal common duct, and a normal pancreatic duct.

What is it? Malignant, but lucky: probably cholangiocarcinoma at the lower end of the common duct. He could be cured with a pancreatoduodenectomy (Whipple operation).

Management. Get brushings of the common duct for cytologic diagnosis.

55. A 64-year-old woman presents with progressive jaundice, which she first noticed 2 weeks ago. She has a total bilirubin of 12, with 8 direct and 4 indirect, and minimally elevated transaminases. The alkaline phosphatase is about 10 times the upper limit of normal. She is otherwise asymptomatic, but is found to be slightly anemic and to have positive occult blood in the stool. A sonogram shows dilated intrahepatic ducts, dilated extrahepatic ducts, and a very distended, thin-walled gallbladder.

What is it? Again malignant, but also lucky. The coincidence of slowly bleeding into the GI tract at the same time that she develops obstructive jaundice points to an ampullary carcinoma, another malignancy that can be cured with radical surgery.

Management. Endoscopy with U/S assistance.

56. A 56-year-old man presents with progressive jaundice, which he first noticed 6 weeks ago. He has a total bilirubin of 22, with 16 direct and 6 indirect, and minimally elevated transaminases. The alkaline phosphatase is about 8 times the upper limit of normal. He has lost 20 pounds over the past 2 months, and has a persistent, nagging mild pain deep into his epigastrium and in the upper back. His sister died at age 44 from a cancer of the pancreas. A sonogram shows dilated intrahepatic ducts, dilated extrahepatic ducts, and a very distended, thin-walled gallbladder.

What is it? Bad news. Cancer of the head of the pancreas. Terrible prognosis.

Diagnosis. Nowadays, endoscopic U/S has become a standard part of the pancreatic head mass work-up. U/S-guided FNAC is increasingly being used for diagnosis. Endoscopic retrograde cholangiopancreatography (ERCP) has a limited role in placing stents to decompress the bile duct if total bilirubin is >20.

Gallbladder

57. A white, obese 40-year-old mother of 5 children gives a history of repeated episodes of right upper quadrant abdominal pain brought about by the ingestion of fatty foods, and relieved by the administration of anticholinergic medications. The pain is colicky, radiates to the right shoulder and around to the back, and is accompanied by nausea and occasional vomiting. Physical examination is unremarkable.

What is it? Gallstones, with biliary colic.

Management. Sonogram. Elective cholecystectomy will follow.

58. A 43-year-old obese mother of 6 children has severe right upper quadrant abdominal pain that began 6 hours ago. The pain was colicky at first, radiated to the right shoulder and around toward the back, and was accompanied by nausea and vomiting. For the past 2 hours the pain has been constant. She has tenderness to deep palpation, muscle guarding, and rebound in the right upper quadrant. Her temperature is 101° F, and WBC count 12,000. Liver function tests are normal.

What is it? If you are alert, you will recognize the picture of acute cholecystitis. A similar vignette was presented in the acute abdomen section. It is repeated here to contrast it with the next one. She will get a cholecystectomy, as previously mentioned.

59. A 73-year-old obese mother of 6 children has severe right upper quadrant abdominal pain that began 3 days ago. The pain was colicky at first but has been constant for the past 2.5 days. She has tenderness to deep palpation, muscle guarding, and rebound in the right upper quadrant. She has temperature spikes of 104 and 105°F, with chills. WBC count is 22,000, with a shift to the left. Her bilirubin is 5, and she has an alkaline phosphatase of 2,000 (~20x normal).

What is it? Acute ascending cholangitis.

Diagnosis. The diagnosis is already clear. Sonogram might confirm dilated ducts.

Management. This is an emergency, and many things will be needed at once. The therapy is based on IV antibiotics plus emergency decompression of the biliary tract. To achieve the latter, ERCP is the first choice, but percutaneous transhepatic cholangiogram (PTC) is another option (and surgery is a distant third choice).

60. A white, obese 40-year-old mother of 5 children gives a history of repeated episodes of right upper quadrant abdominal pain brought about by the ingestion of fatty foods, and relieved by the administration of anticholinergic medications. The pain is colicky, radiates to the right shoulder and around to the back, and is accompanied by nausea and occasional vomiting. This time she had a shaking chill with the colicky pain, and the pain lasted longer than usual. She has mild tenderness to palpation in the epigastrium and right upper quadrant. Laboratory determinations show a bilirubin of 3.5, an alkaline phosphatase 5 times normal, and serum lipase 3 times normal value.

What is it? She passed a common duct stone and had a transient episode of cholangitis (the shaking chill, the high phosphatase) and a bit of biliary pancreatitis (the high amylase).

Management. As in many of these cases, start with sonogram. It will confirm the diagnosis of gallstones. If she continues to get well, elective cholecystectomy will follow. If she deteriorates, she may have the stone still impacted at the ampulla of Vater, and may need ERCP and sphincterotomy to extract it.

Pancreas

61. A 33-year-old alcoholic man shows up in the ED with epigastric and midabdominal pain that began 12 hours ago shortly after the ingestion of a large meal. The pain is constant and very severe, and radiates straight through to the back. He vomited twice early on, but since then has continued to have retching. He has tenderness and some muscle guarding in the upper abdomen, is afebrile, and has mild tachycardia. Serum lipase is 1,200, and his hematocrit is 52%.

What is it? Acute pancreatitis.

Management. Put the pancreas at rest: NPO, NG suction, IV fluids.

62. A 56-year-old alcoholic man is admitted with a clinical picture of acute upper abdominal pain. The pain is constant, radiates straight through the back, and is extremely severe. He has a serum amylase of 800, a hematocrit of 40%, WBC count of 18,000, blood glucose of 150 mg/dl, and serum calcium of 6.5. He is given IV fluids and kept NPO with NG suction. By the next morning, his hematocrit has dropped to 30%, the serum calcium has remained below 7 despite calcium administration, his blood urea nitrogen (BUN) has gone up to 32, and he has developed metabolic acidosis and a low arterial Po2.

What is it? He has acute severe pancreatitis. In fact, he is in deep trouble, with at least 8 of Ranson's criteria predicting 80 to 100% mortality.

Management. Very intensive support will be needed, but the common pathway to death from complications of hemorrhagic pancreatitis frequently is by way of pancreatic abscesses that need to be drained as soon as they appear. Thus serial CT scans will be required. In very select patients there is a role for necrosectomy to get rid of dead pancreatic tissue.

63. A 57-year-old alcoholic man is being treated for acute hemorrhagic pancreatitis. He was in the ICU for 1 week, required chest tubes for pleural effusion, and was on a respirator for several days, but eventually improved enough to be transferred to the floor. Two weeks after the onset of the disease, he begins to spike fever and to demonstrate leukocytosis. He looks septic.

What is it? Pancreatic abscess.

Diagnosis. CT scan.

Management. Drainage and appropriate antibiotics.

64. A 49-year-old alcoholic man presents with ill-defined upper abdominal discomfort and early satiety. On physical examination he has a large epigastric mass that is deep within the abdomen and actually hard to define. He was discharged from the hospital 5 weeks ago, after successful treatment for acute pancreatitis.

65. A 55-year-old woman presents with vague upper abdominal discomfort, early satiety, and a large but ill-defined epigastric mass. Five weeks ago she was involved in an automobile accident in which she hit the upper abdomen against the steering wheel.

What is it? The 2 presentations of pancreatic pseudocyst.

Management. You could diagnose it on the cheap with a sonogram, but CT scan is probably the best choice. Small cysts (<6 cm) which have not been present too long (<6 weeks) can be watched for spontaneous resolution. Bigger or older cysts could have serious complications (obstruction, infection, bleeding) and they need intervention. Internal surgical derivation (cystogastrostomy or cystojejunostomy) is the standard surgical treatment. Radiologically guided external drainage is option, often used for infected pseudocysts. The latest and very appealing (if technically feasible) is endoscopic cystogastrostomy, which can only be done for cysts with a completely liquid content without debris.

66. A disheveled, malnourished individual shows up in the ED requesting medication for pain. He smells of alcohol and complains bitterly of constant epigastric pain radiating straight through to the back which he says he has had for several years. He has diabetes, steatorrhea, and calcifications in the upper abdomen in a plain x-ray.

What is it? Chronic pancreatitis.

Management. There is little that can be done for a patient like this. Stopping the alcoholic intake is the first step (easier said than done). Replacement of pancreatic enzymes and control of the diabetes are obvious needs. Sometimes the pancreatic enzymes will relieve the pain, but if they do not, the pain will be very difficult to eradicate. Various operations can be performed that would be guided by the anatomy of the pancreatic ducts; thus, if forced to go to further diagnostic tests, pick ERCP.

Hernias

67. A 9-month-old baby girl is brought in because she has an umbilical hernia. The defect is 1 cm in diameter, and the contents are freely reducible.

Although we routinely recommend elective surgical repair of all hernias (to prevent the ghastly complication of strangulation), there are some exceptions. This is one. Umbilical hernias in children age <5 years may still close spontaneously. Only observation is needed here. If present at age 5 years, repair is usually performed.

68. An 18-year-old man has a routine physical examination as part of his college registration, and the examination reveals that he has a right inguinal hernia. The external inguinal ring is about 2.5 cm in diameter, and a hernial bulge can be easily seen and felt going down into his scrotum when he is asked to strain. He is completely asymptomatic and was not even aware of the presence of the hernia.

Elective surgical repair is in order. Even though he is asymptomatic, he should not be exposed to the risk of bowel strangulation. They will not ask you about specific technical details. The hernia is probably indirect. All routine unilateral first-time hernias can be repaired by open or laparoscopic approach with a mesh. Laparoscopy is often favored for repair of recurrent inguinal, bilateral inguinal, and incisional hernias.

69. A 72-year-old farmer is forced by his insurance company to have a physical examination to be issued a life insurance policy. He has been healthy all his life, and "has never been to the doctor." At the examination it is found that he has a large, left inguinal hernia that reaches down into the scrotum. Bowel sounds can be easily heard over it. The hernia is not reducible, and he says that many years ago he used to be able to "push it back," but for the last 10 or 20 years he has not been able to do so.

A hernia that cannot be pushed back in (reduced) is incarcerated, and one that has compromised blood supply is strangulated. The latter is an emergency. The former is also an emergency if the irreducible state is of new onset, because one does not want to wait for overt signs of dead or compromised bowel before operating. But if he has been this way for 10 or 20 years, obviously the bowel is alive and well. Elective repair is still indicated, before he runs out of good luck and gets into trouble.

DISEASES OF THE BREAST

1. An 18-year-old woman has a firm, rubbery mass in the left breast that moves easily with palpation.

What is it? Fibroadenoma.

Management. The underlying concern in all breast masses is cancer, and the best predictor of the likelihood of malignancy is age. At age 18, the chances of malignancy are very remote; thus, the least invasive way to make the diagnosis is, in order, sonogram or needle biopsy. Sonogram is diagnostic for fibroadenomas. Reassurance alone would not be a good choice! Do not order a mammogram either. At age 18, mammograms are virtually useless (breast too dense). Sonogram is the only imaging technique suitable for the very young breast. Once diagnosis is confirmed, excision is optional.

2. A 14-year-old girl has a firm, movable, rubbery mass in her left breast that was first noticed 1 year ago and has since grown to be about 6 cm in diameter.

What is it? Giant juvenile fibroadenoma.

Management. At age 14 chances of cancer are virtually zero. That avenue does not have to be explored. But the rapid growth requires resection to avoid cosmetic deformity.

3. A 37-year-old woman has a 12- × 10- × 7-cm mass in her left breast. It has been present for 7 years, and has been slowly growing to its present size. The mass—firm, rubbery, completely movable—is not attached to chest wall or to overlying skin. There are no palpable axillary nodes.

What is it? Cystosarcoma phyllodes, a benign condition that can turn into an outright malignant sarcoma.

Management. After tissue diagnosis, proceed with margin-free resection.

4. A 35-year-old woman has a 10-year history of tenderness in both breasts, related to her menstrual cycle, with multiple lumps on both breasts that seem to "come and go" at different times in the menstrual cycle. She now has a firm, round, 2-cm mass that has not gone away for 6 weeks.

What is it? Palpable cyst in fibrocystic disease (cystic mastitis, mammary dysplasia).

Management. Start with a mammogram to evaluate for any lesions suspicious for malignancy. An ultrasound is also helpful in evaluating the persistent mass. A cyst is the most likely candidate. Once confirmed by ultrasound, aspiration of the cyst can be performed for symptom relief. Otherwise, a simple cyst can be left alone. (Note: if aspiration is performed for symptom relief, it is important to understand that this is not the same as FNA biopsy—this is aspiration of fluid to empty a cyst, not aspiration of a solid mass to get cells for diagnosis). If the mass goes away and the fluid aspirated is clear, that's all. If, however, the fluid is bloody, it goes to cytology. If the mass does not go away or recurs multiple times, she needs a biopsy.

5. A 34-year-old woman has been having bloody discharge from the right nipple, on and off for several months. There are no palpable masses.

What is it? Intraductal papilloma.

Management. Although cancer is a concern with bloody nipple discharge, the most common cause of this complaint happens to be benign intraductal papilloma. The concern over cancer must be ruled out; the way to detect cancer that is not palpable is with mammogram. That should be the first choice. If negative, one may still wish to find and resect the intraductal papilloma to provide symptomatic relief and further exclude malignancy given the bloody discharge. Resection can be guided by galactogram, sonogram, or done as a retroareolar exploration.

6. A 26-year-old lactating mother has cracks in the nipple and develops a fluctuating, red, hot, tender mass in the breast, along with fever and leukocytosis.

What is it? Sounds like an abscess—and in this setting it is. Breast feeding is a common cause of breast abscess. In anybody else, a breast abscess is a cancer until proven otherwise.

Management. There would be low yield to obtaining a mammogram in this case (age, lactation, low-risk presentation for cancer). Drainage is the treatment for all abscesses, this one included. Ultrasound-guided needle drainage is preferred in lactating women, since a formal incision and drainage carries a higher risk of developing a persistent milk fistula in the lactating breast.

7. A 49-year-old woman has a firm, 2-cm mass in the right breast, which has been present for 3 months.

What is it? This could be anything. Age is the best determinant for risk for cancer of the breast. If she had been 72, you go for cancer. At 22, you favor benign.

Management. Mammogram to assess the palpable mass and to explore for other non-palpable lesions (don't want to miss anything). An ultrasound of the mass would also be helpful. Then, multiple core biopsies of the known 2-cm mass are needed.

8. A 34-year-old woman in month 5 of pregnancy reports a 3-cm firm, ill-defined mass in her right breast that has been present and growing for 3 months.

The diagnosis of possible breast cancer in the pregnant patient is done the same way as if she had not been pregnant. Yes, you can do the mammogram (with appropriate fetal shielding used) and appropriate biopsies; but the radiologist will probably use sonogram to guide the biopsies, and no, you do not need to terminate the pregnancy.

9. A 69-year-old woman has a 4-cm hard mass in the right breast with ill-defined borders, movable from the chest wall but not movable within the breast. The skin overlying the mass is retracted and has an "orange peel" appearance.

10. A 69-year-old woman has a 4-cm hard mass in the right breast under the nipple and areola with ill-defined borders, movable from the chest wall but not movable within the breast. The nipple became retracted 6 months ago.

11. A 72-year-old woman has a red, swollen breast. The skin over the area looks like orange peel. She is not particularly tender, and it is debatable whether the area is hot or not. She has no fever or leukocytosis.

12. A 62-year-old woman has an eczematoid lesion in the areola. It has been present for 3 months, and it looks to her like "some kind of skin condition" that has not improved or gone away with a variety of lotions and ointments.

These are all classic presentations of breast cancer. The hard masses are likely invasive breast adenocarcinoma. The red, orange peel skin is likely inflammatory breast cancer, and the eczematoid areolar lesion is likely Paget's disease of the breast (a rare form of breast cancer). They all need mammograms for further evaluation and multiple core biopsies of suspicious breast lesions. The suspicious skin lesions (e.g. orange peel, eczematoid) can be confirmed with dermal punch biopsies.

13. A 42-year-old woman hits her breast with a broom handle while doing her housework. She noticed a lump in that area at the time, and 1 week later the lump is still there. She has a 3-cm hard mass deep inside the affected breast, and some superficial ecchymosis over the area.

What is it? This is a classic trap for the unwary. It is cancer until proven otherwise. Trauma often brings the area to the attention of the patient—but is not the cause of the lump. Proceed as with the others.

14. A 58-year-old woman discovers a mass in her right axilla. She has a discrete, hard, movable, 2-cm mass. Physical examination of her breast is negative, and she has no enlarged lymph nodes elsewhere.

What is it? A tough one, but another potential presentation for cancer of the breast. It could be lymphoma but also may be lymph node metastasis from an occult primary. She needs a mammogram (we are now looking for an occult primary in the breast) and possible U/S. The node will eventually have to be biopsied. MRI of the breast is now in the work-up for occult primary breast cancer, as many are lobular cancers which are not always visualized by mammogram or even U/S.

> 15. A 60-year-old woman has a routine, screening mammogram. The radiologist reports an irregular area of increased density, with fine microcalcifications, that was not present 2 years ago on a previous mammogram.

Management. You will not be asked to read difficult x-rays (particularly mammograms), but you should recognize the description of a malignant radiologic image—which this one is. Thus, we go back to our old issue: we need tissue diagnosis. The mammographer will obtain multiple core biopsies.

> 16. A 44-year-old woman has a 2-cm palpable mass in the upper outer quadrant of her right breast. A core biopsy shows infiltrating ductal carcinoma. The mass is freely movable, and her breast is of normal, rather generous size. She has no palpable axillary nodes, and the mammogram showed no other lesions.

Treatment of operable breast cancer begins (but does not end) with surgery. With a small tumor far away from the nipple, the standard option is partial mastectomy (lumpectomy) and axillary node sampling (i.e. sentinel node biopsy) to help determine the need for adjuvant systemic therapy. Why go after the axillary nodes when they are not palpable? Because palpation is notoriously inaccurate in detecting microscopic metastasis to the lymph nodes which may be present in the early stages of an invasive breast cancer. Afterward, radiation therapy is typically given to the breast (otherwise, lumpectomy would have an unacceptably high rate of local recurrence).

> 17. A 62-year-old woman has a 4-cm hard mass under the nipple and areola of her smallish left breast. A core biopsy has diagnosed infiltrating ductal carcinoma. There are no palpable axillary nodes. The mammogram shows extensive associated branching calcifications thought to represent DCIS.

Lumpectomy is an ideal option when the tumor is small (in relation to the size of the breast), is located where most of the breast can be spared, and can be performed in a way that maintains the cosmetic appearance of the breast. A total mastectomy (also called simple mastectomy) is the choice here given the extent of disease. If necessary, a biopsy can be performed of the suspicious calcifications to confirm malignancy if there is any doubt. Axillary sampling of sentinel nodes is also required (i.e. sentinel node biopsy if no palpable nodes).

Radiation is typically not needed when the whole breast is removed unless in rare circumstances where the mass is very large (e.g., ≥5 cm) or if the lymph nodes contain metastasis. The old (unmodified) radical mastectomy is no longer done.

18. A 44-year-old woman has a 2-cm palpable mass in the upper outer quadrant of her right breast. A core biopsy shows lobular cancer.

19. A 44-year-old woman has a 2-cm palpable mass in the upper outer quadrant of her right breast. A core biopsy shows medullary cancer of the breast.

If you see on the exam breast cancers that are not the standard infiltrating ductal carcinoma, here are the rules: lobular has a higher incidence of bilaterality (but not enough to justify bilateral mastectomy). Almost all the other variants of invasive cancer have a little better prognosis than infiltrating ductal, and they are all treated the same way anyway.

20. A 52-year-old woman has a suspicious area on mammogram. Multiple radiologically guided core biopsies show ductal carcinoma in situ.

No axillary sampling is needed if a lumpectomy is being performed. Lumpectomy and radiation should be offered in cases of limited DCIS. If there are multicentric lesions all over the breast, total mastectomy (also called simple mastectomy) is needed. Sentinel node biopsy should be done in the event that invasive carcinoma is found on the mastectomy pathology, since you cannot go back to do a sentinel node biopsy once the breast has been removed.

21. A 32-year-old woman in the seventh month of pregnancy is found to have a 2-cm mass in her left breast. Mammogram shows no other lesions, and core biopsy reveals infiltrating ductal carcinoma.

Again, pregnancy imposes very few limitations on our handling of breast cancer. The only no-no's are: no radiation therapy during the pregnancy, and no chemotherapy during the first trimester. Termination of the pregnancy is not needed.

22. A 44-year-old woman arrives in the ED because she is "bleeding from the breast." Physical examination shows a huge, fungating, ulcerated mass occupying the entire right breast, and firmly attached to the chest wall. The patient maintains that the mass has been present for only "a few weeks," but a relative indicates that it has been there at least 2 years, maybe longer.

An all-too-frequent tragic case of neglect and denial. Obviously, this is a far advanced cancer of the breast. Tissue diagnosis is still needed, and either a core or an incisional biopsy is in order, but the likely question here is what to do next. This is inoperable, and incurable as well, but palliation can be offered. Chemotherapy (or hormone therapy if the tumor is hormone receptor positive) may be considered in the first line of treatment, perhaps accompanied by radiation. In many cases the tumor will shrink enough to become operable for palliative surgery.

23. A 37-year-old woman has a lumpectomy and axillary sentinel node biopsy for a 3-cm infiltrating ductal carcinoma. The pathologist reports clear surgical margins and metastatic cancer in both of the sentinel nodes that were removed. The tumor is positive for estrogen and progesterone receptors.

Very rarely is surgery alone sufficient to cure breast cancer. Many patients require subsequent adjuvant systemic therapy. The need for it is underscored by the finding of involved axillary nodes. Chemotherapy is indicated here, followed by radiation (because she had a lumpectomy) and finally, hormonal therapy, which, given her age, should be tamoxifen. According to the results of the American College of Surgeons Oncology Group Z0011 trial, patients undergoing lumpectomy and radiation who have T1-T2 invasive breast cancer, no palpable adenopathy, and only 1–2 sentinel lymph nodes containing limited metastases may safely avoid an axillary dissection.

24. A 66-year-old woman has a total mastectomy for infiltrating ductal carcinoma of the breast. The pathologist reports that the tumor measures 1 cm in diameter and that 1 of 2 sentinel nodes removed are positive for metastasis. The tumor is estrogen and progesterone receptor positive.

The hormonal therapy of choice for post-menopausal women is an aromatase inhibitor (e.g., anastrazole). This may follow chemotherapy depending on the specific tumor features of the case (including possible Oncotype DX testing). As a general rule, all invasive cancers should be treated locally by surgery/radiation therapy and systemically by chemo/hormonal therapy (exceptions are very small, low-risk breast cancers, typically in elderly women, which may not require any adjuvant systemic therapy).

25. A 44-year-old woman complains bitterly of severe headaches that have been present for several weeks and have not responded to the usual over-the-counter headache remedies. She is 2 years post-op from MRM for T3 N2 M0 cancer of the breast, and she had several courses of post-op chemotherapy, which she eventually discontinued because of the side effects.

A classic: severe headache in someone who a few years ago had extensive cancer of the breast means brain metastases until proven otherwise. Don't get hung up on the TNM classification; if the numbers are not 1 for the tumor and 0 for the nodes and metastases, the tumor is bad. Do MRI of the brain and use high-dose steroids and radiation.

26. A 39-year-old woman completed her last course of postoperative adjuvant chemotherapy for breast cancer 6 months ago. She comes to the clinic complaining of constant back pain for about 3 weeks. She is tender to palpation over 2 well-circumscribed areas in the thoracic and lumbar spine.

A variation on the above theme. Now it is bone metastases, instead of brain metastases—at least until proven otherwise. What do you do? MRI for diagnosis. Local radiation to the metastases may help, and a variety of orthopedic supports can be used to prevent collapse of the vertebral bodies and pedicles.

DISEASES OF THE ENDOCRINE SYSTEM

1. A 62-year-old woman was drinking her morning cup of coffee at the same time she was applying her makeup, and she noticed in the mirror that there was a lump in the lower part of the neck, visible when she swallowed. She consults you for this, and on physical examination you ascertain that she indeed has a prominent, 2-cm mass on the left lobe of her thyroid as well as 2 smaller masses on the right lobe. They are all soft, and she has no palpable lymph nodes in the neck.

Management. Most thyroid nodules are benign, and surgical removal to ascertain the diagnosis is a big operation—thus surgery has to be reserved for selected cases. Worrisome features include: young, male, single nodule, history of radiation to the neck, solid mass on sonogram, and cold nodule on scan. In centers with sufficient experience, the last 2 tests are omitted in preference for FNA and cytology. This case does not sound malignant, but you cannot be sure. If given the option among the answers, go for the FNA.

2. A 21-year-old man is found on a routine physical examination to have a single, 2-cm nodule in the thyroid gland. His thyroid function tests are normal. An FNA is read as indeterminate.

Management. Surgery is done for the FNAs that are read as malignant and those that are indeterminate.

3. A 32-year-old woman has a thyroid lobectomy done for a 2-cm mass that had been reported on a FNA as a "follicular neoplasm, not otherwise specified." The specimen is given for frozen section to a pathologist with a great deal of experience in thyroid disease and in the reading of frozen sections. The intraoperative diagnosis is follicular cancer.

Management. A total thyroidectomy should be completed.

4. An automated blood chemistry panel done during the course of a routine medical examination indicates that an asymptomatic patient has a serum calcium of 12.1 in a lab where the upper limit of normal is 9.5. Repeated determinations are consistently between 10.5 and 12.6. Serum phosphorus is low.

What is it? Parathyroid adenoma.

Diagnosis. Had this question been written 20 years ago, the vignette would have described a patient with a disease of "stones and bones and abdominal groans," and you would have cleverly asked for a serum calcium as your first test. Today most parathyroid adenomas are identified when they are still asymptomatic, because of the widespread use of automated blood chemistry panels. Across the board, most cases of hypercalcemia are caused by metastatic cancer, but that would not be the case on asymptomatic people. Your next move here is parathyroid hormone (PTH) determination and sestamibi scan to localize the adenoma. Surgery will follow.

5. A 32-year-old woman is admitted to the psychiatry unit because of wild mood swings. She is found to be hypertensive and diabetic and to have osteoporosis. (She had not been aware of such diagnosis beforehand.) It is also ascertained that she has been amenorrheic and shaving for the past couple of years. She has gross centripetal obesity, with moon facies and buffalo hump, and thin, bruised extremities. A picture from 3 years ago shows a person of very different, more normal appearance.

What is it? Cushing's syndrome. The appearance is so typical that you will probably be given before and after photographs on the exam, with a brief vignette. The presenting symptom may be any one of those listed.

Diagnosis. Start with the overnight dose dexamethasone suppression test. If she suppresses at a low dose, she is an obese, hairy woman, but she does not have the disease. If she does not suppress at the low dose, verify that 24-hour urine-free cortisol is elevated, and then go to high-dose suppression tests. If she suppresses at a high dose, do an MRI of the head looking for the pituitary microadenoma, which will be removed by the transnasal, trans-sphenoidal route. If she does not suppress at the higher dose, do a CT or MRI of adrenals looking for the adenoma there.

6. A 28-year-old woman has virulent peptic ulcer disease. Extensive medical management including eradication of *Helicobacter pylori* fails to heal her ulcers. She has several duodenal ulcers in the first and second portions of the duodenum. She has watery diarrhea.

What is it? Gastrinoma (Zollinger-Ellison syndrome).

Diagnosis. Start by measuring serum gastrin. If the value is not clearly normal or abnormal, a secretin stimulation test is added. Later, do CT scans (with vascular and GI contrast) of the pancreas and nearby area to find the tumor, and then do surgery to remove it.

7. A second-year medical student is hospitalized for a neurologic workup for a seizure disorder of recent onset. During one of the convulsions, it is determined that his blood sugar is extremely low. Further workup shows that he has high levels of insulin in the blood with low levels of C-peptide.

What is it? Exogenous administration of insulin. If the C-peptide had been high along with the insulin level, the diagnosis would have been insulinoma. Had it been a baby with high insulin level and low blood sugar, it would have been nesidioblastosis.

Management. In this case, psychiatric evaluation and counseling (he is faking the disease to avoid taking the USMLE). If it had been insulinoma, CT scan (with vascular and GI contrast) looking for the tumor in the pancreas, and subsequent surgical removal.

8. A 48-year-old woman has had severe, migratory necrolytic dermatitis for several years, unresponsive to all kinds of "herbs and unguents." She is thin and has mild stomatitis and mild diabetes mellitus.

What is it? Glucagonoma.

Diagnosis. Determine glucagon levels. Eventually CT scan (with vascular and GI contrast) looking for the tumor in the pancreas. Surgery will follow. If inoperable, somatostatin can help symptomatically, and streptozocin is the indicated chemotherapeutic agent.

SURGICAL HYPERTENSION

1. A 45-year-old woman comes into your office for a regular checkup. On repeated determinations you confirm the fact that she is hypertensive. When she was in your office 3 years ago, her BP was normal. Laboratory studies at this time show a serum sodium of 144 mEq/L, a serum bicarbonate of 28 mEq/L, and a serum potassium concentration of 2.1 mEq/L. The woman is taking no medications of any kind.

What is it? Hyperaldosteronism. Possibly adenoma.

Diagnosis. Start with determination of aldosterone and renin levels. If confirmatory (aldosterone high, renin low), proceed with determinations lying down and sitting up to differentiate hyperplasia (appropriate response to postural changes—not surgical) from adenoma (no response or wrong response to postural changes—surgical). Treat the first with Aldactone. Pursue the second with imaging studies (CT or MRI) and surgery.

2. A thin, hyperactive 38-year-old woman is frustrated by the inability of her physicians to help her. She has episodes of severe pounding headache, with palpitations, profuse perspiration, and pallor, but by the time she gets to her doctor's office she checks out normal in every respect. In addition, she has paroxismal hypertension.

What is it? Suspect pheochromocytoma.

Diagnosis. The most sensitive test is the 24-hour urinary metanephrine test (90% effective). The vanillylmandelic acid (VMA) test is next best, at 80% effective. Follow with CT scan of adrenal glands. Surgery will eventually be done, with careful pharmacologic preparation with alpha-blockers.

3. A 17-year-old man is found to have a BP of 190 over 115. This is checked repeatedly in both arms, and it is always found to be elevated, but when checked in the legs it is found to be normal.

What is it? Coarctation of the aorta.

Diagnosis. Start with a chest x-ray, looking for scalloping of the ribs. Then CTA and ultimately surgery.

4. A 23-year-old woman has had severe hypertension for 2 years, and she does not respond well to the usual medical treatment for that condition. A bruit can be faintly heard over her upper abdomen.

5. A 72-year-old man with multiple manifestations of arteriosclerotic occlusive disease has hypertension of relatively recent onset and refractory to the usual medical therapy. He has a faint bruit over the upper abdomen.

What is it? Two examples of renovascular hypertension; the first one caused by fibromuscular dysplasia, the second one secondary to arteriosclerosis.

Diagnosis. Start with Duplex scanning of the renal vessels. CT angio may also be helpful.

Management. Once the diagnosis has been made, the decision for therapy is easy in the young woman: she has many years of potential life, and her hypertension must be cured. Angiographic balloon dilation with stenting is the first choice, surgery the other alternative.

In the elderly man the decision is far more complex. Treatment of the renovascular hypertension makes sense only if other manifestations of the arteriosclerosis are not going to kill him first.

Pediatric Surgery 5

AT BIRTH—THE FIRST 24 HOURS

1. Within 8 hours after birth, it is noted that a baby has excessive salivation. A small, soft NG tube is inserted, and the baby is taken to x-ray to have a "babygram" done. The film shows the tube coiled back on itself in the upper chest. There is air in the GI tract.

What is it? Tracheoesophageal (TE) fistula, the most common type, with proximal blind esophageal pouch and distal TE fistula.

Management. First, rule out the associated anomalies (VACTER: vertebral, anal, cardiac, TE, and renal/radial). The vertebral and radial will be seen in the same x-ray you already took, you need echocardiogram for the heart, sonogram for the kidneys, and physical examination for the anus. Then off to surgery.

2. A newborn baby is found on physical examination to have an imperforate anus.

Management. This is part of the VACTER group, so rule out the other components. For the anal problem, if there is a fistula to the vagina or perineum, repair can be safely done later, as the GI tract is not obstructed. If there is no fistula, one has to ascertain the level of the blind pouch. This is done with an x-ray while holding the baby upside down, with a metal marker taped to the anal dimple. Low imperforate anus can be corrected with a very simple operation. High imperforate anus needs a colostomy, and repair at a later date.

3. A newborn baby is found to be tachypneic, cyanotic, and grunting. The abdomen is scaphoid, and there are bowel sounds heard over the left chest. An x-ray confirms that there is bowel in the left thorax. Shortly thereafter, the baby develops significant hypoxia and acidosis.

What is it? Congenital diaphragmatic hernia.

Management. The main problem is the hypoplastic lung. It is better to wait 36 to 48 hours to do surgery to allow transition from fetal circulation to newborn circulation. Meanwhile, the trick is to keep the child alive with endotracheal intubation, low-pressure hyperventilation (careful not to blow up the other lung), sedation, and NG suction.

4. At the time of birth, it is noted that a child has a large abdominal wall defect to the right of the umbilicus. There is a normal cord, but protruding from the defect is a matted mass of angry-looking edematous bowel loops.

5. A newborn baby is noted to have a shiny, thin, membranous sac at the base of the umbilical cord (the cord goes to the sac, not to the baby). Inside the sac, one can see part of the liver and loops of normal bowel.

What is it? The first vignette is gastroschisis, the second one omphalocele. Medical school professors love to emphasize differential diagnoses of somewhat similar problems. Chances are all you'll be expected to do is to identify the correct one.

Management. Intuitive. You've got to get those intestines back into the belly, and the technical details are best left to the pediatric surgeons. They will be on the lookout for atresias (which babies with gastroschisis can have) or multiple defects (which are seen with omphalocele), and they will close small defects directly. Very often, however, the defects are large, most of the bowel is outside the abdomen, and there is no room to "push it in." In those cases a silicon "silo" is used to house the bowel and gradually return it to the abdomen. The baby with gastroschisis will also need vascular access for IV nutrition (the angry bowel will not work for about 1 month).

6. A newborn is noted to have a moist medallion of mucosae occupying the lower abdominal wall, above the pubis and below the umbilicus. It is clear that urine is constantly bathing this congenital anomaly.

What is it? Exstrophy of the urinary bladder.

What's the point of the vignette? These are very rare anomalies that only very highly specialized centers can repair. The problem is that unless the repair is done within the first 48 hours, it will not have a good chance to succeed. It takes time to arrange for transfer of a newborn baby to a distant city. If a day or 2 are wasted before arrangements are made, it will be too late.

7. Half an hour after the first feed, a baby vomits greenish fluid. The mother had polyhydramnios, and the baby has Down syndrome. X-ray shows a "double bubble sign": a large air-fluid level in the stomach, and a smaller one in the first portion of the duodenum. There is no gas in the rest of the bowel.

What is it? It can be 2 things, but first some general points. Kids vomit, burp, and regurgitate all the time (ask any parent), but the innocent vomit is clear-whitish. Green vomiting in the newborn is bad news. It means something serious. The 2 conditions that this could be are duodenal atresia and annular pancreas. Malrotation is also possible, but I expect that one to be presented to you as in the next vignette.

Management. With complete obstruction, surgery will be needed, but these kids have lots of other congenital anomalies, look for them first.

8. Half an hour after the first feed, a baby vomits greenish fluid. X-ray shows a "double-bubble sign": a large air-fluid level in the stomach and a smaller one in the first portion of the duodenum. There is air in the distal bowel, beyond the duodenum, in loops that are not distended.

What is it? Now you have 3 choices: it could be an incomplete obstruction from duodenal stenosis or annular pancreas, or it could be malrotation.

Management. If you are dealing with incomplete obstruction, you have time to do what's needed, i.e., it is a lesser emergency. But if it is malrotation the bowel could twist and die, so that would be a super-emergency. How can you tell? A contrast enema is safe but not always diagnostic. An upper GI study is riskier but more reliable.

9. A newborn baby has repeated green vomiting during the first day of life, and does not pass any meconium. Except for abdominal distention, the baby is otherwise normal. X-ray shows multiple air-fluid levels and distended loops of bowel.

What is it? Intestinal atresia.

Management. This one is caused by a vascular accident in utero; thus, there are no other congenital anomalies to look for, but there may be multiple points of atresia.

A FEW DAYS OLD TO THE FIRST 2 MONTHS OF LIFE

1. A very premature baby develops feeding intolerance, abdominal distention, and a rapidly dropping platelet count. The baby is 4 days old, and was treated with indomethacin for a patent ductus arteriosus.

What is it? Necrotizing enterocolitis.

Management. Stop all feedings, broad-spectrum antibiotics, IV fluids/nutrition. Surgical intervention may be needed if the baby develops abdominal wall erythema, air in the portal vein, or pneumoperitoneum.

2. A 3-day-old, full-term baby is brought in because of feeding intolerance and bilious vomiting. X-ray shows multiple dilated loops of small bowel and a ground-glass appearance in the lower abdomen. The mother has cystic fibrosis.

What is it? Meconium ileus.

Management. Gastrografin enema may be both diagnostic and therapeutic, so it is the obvious first choice. If unsuccessful, surgery may be needed. The baby has cystic fibrosis, and management of the other manifestations of the disease will also be needed.

3. A 3-week-old baby has had "trouble feeding" and is not quite growing well. He now has bilious vomiting and is brought in for evaluation. X-ray shows a classic "double bubble," along with normal-looking gas pattern in the rest of the bowel.

What is it? Malrotation. The vignette is repeated here because it can show up at any time within the first few weeks of life. Proceed with urgent diagnostic studies.

4. A 3-week-old first-born, full-term baby boy began to vomit 3 days ago. The vomiting is projectile, has no bile in it, and follows each feeding, and the baby is hungry and eager to eat again after he vomits. He looks somewhat dehydrated and has visible gastric peristaltic waves and a palpable "olive size" mass in the right upper quadrant.

What is it? Hypertrophic pyloric stenosis.

Management. Check electrolytes; hypokalemic, hypochloremic metabolic alkalosis may have developed. Correct it, rehydrate, and do a pyloromyotomy.

5. An 8-week-old baby is brought in because of persistent, progressively increasing jaundice. The bilirubin is significantly elevated, and about 2/3 of it is conjugated, direct bilirubin. Serology is negative for hepatitis, and sweat test is normal.

What is it? Biliary atresia.

Management. HIDA scan after 1 week of phenobarbital is the best test. Surgical derivation will be tried, but 2/3 of these children end up with liver transplant.

6. A 2-month-old baby boy is brought in because of chronic constipation. He has abdominal distention, and plain x-rays show gas in dilated loops of bowel throughout the abdomen. Rectal examination is followed by explosive expulsion of stool and flatus, with remarkable improvement of the distention.

What is it? Hirschsprung disease (aganglionic megacolon).

Diagnosis. Barium enema will define the normal-looking aganglionic distal colon and the abnormal-looking, distended, normal proximal colon; but the diagnosis is established with full thickness biopsy of the rectal mucosa.

LATER IN INFANCY

1. A 9-month-old, chubby, healthy-looking little boy has episodes of colicky abdominal pain that makes him double up and squat. The pain lasts for about 1 minute, and the kid looks perfectly happy and normal until he gets another colic episode. Physical examination shows a vague mass on the right side of the abdomen, an "empty" right lower quadrant, and currant jelly stools.

What is it? Intussusception.

Management. Barium enema or air enema are both diagnostic and therapeutic in most cases. It should be your first choice. If reduction is not achieved radiologically, do surgery.

2. A 1-year-old baby is referred to the University Hospital for treatment of a subdural hematoma. In the admission examination it is noted that the baby has retinal hemorrhages.

3. A 3-year-old girl is brought in for treatment of a fractured humerus. The mother relates that the girl fell from her crib. X-rays show evidence of other older fractures at various stages of healing in different bones.

4. A 1-year-old child is brought in with second-degree burns of both buttocks. The stepfather relates that the child fell into a hot tub.

What is it? These are classic vignettes of child abuse.

Management. Notify the proper authorities.

5. A 7-year-old boy passes a large bloody bowel movement.

What is it? Meckel diverticulum.

Diagnosis. Do a radioisotope scan looking for gastric mucosa in the lower abdomen.

Cardiothoracic Surgery 6

CONGENITAL HEART PROBLEMS

1. A 6-month-old baby has occasional stridor, and episodes of respiratory distress with "crowing" respiration during which he assumes a hyperextended position. The family has also noted mild difficulty in swallowing.

The combination of pressure on the esophagus and pressure on the trachea identifies a vascular ring. Barium swallow will show a typical extrinsic compression from the abnormal vessel. Bronchoscopy confirms the segmental tracheal compression and rules out diffuse tracheomalacia. Surgical repair is done by dividing the smaller of the double aortic arches.

2. A patient who has prosthetic aortic and mitral valves needs extensive dental work.

Antibiotic prophylaxis is needed to protect those valves from bacterial contamination. This is a brief vignette, but you might be expected to remember that these patients need antibiotic prophylaxis for subacute bacterial endocarditis.

3. During a school physical exam, a 12-year-old girl is found to have a heart murmur. She is referred for further evaluation. An alert cardiology fellow recognizes that she indeed has a pulmonary flow systolic murmur, but he also notices that she has a fixed split second heart sound. A history of frequent colds and upper respiratory infections is elicited.

What is it? Atrial septal defect.

Management. Echocardiography to establish the diagnosis. Closure of the defect by open surgery or cardiac catheterization.

4. A 3-month-old boy is hospitalized for "failure to thrive." He has a loud, pansystolic heart murmur best heard at the left sternal border. Chest x-ray shows increased pulmonary vascular markings.

What is it? Ventricular septal defect.

Management. Echocardiography and surgical correction.

5. Because of a heart murmur, an otherwise asymptomatic 3-month-old baby is diagnosed with a small, restrictive ventricular septal defect located low in the muscular septum.

This particular variant has a good chance to close spontaneously within the first 2 or 3 years of life.

6. A 3-day-old premature baby has trouble feeding and pulmonary congestion. Physical examination shows bounding peripheral pulses and a continuous, machinery-like heart murmur. Shortly thereafter, the baby goes into overt heart failure.

What is it? Patent ductus arteriosus.

Management. Echocardiography and surgical closure. In premature infants, surgery is usually reserved for patients who did not close their ductus with indomethacin, but with overt heart failure there is no time to wait. In full-term infants, closure can be achieved with intraluminal coils or surgery.

7. A premature baby girl has mild pulmonary congestion, signs of increased pulmonary blood flow on x-ray, a wide pulse pressure, and a precordial machinery-like murmur. She is not in congestive failure.

Same diagnosis of patent ductus, but with no urgency, and being premature, she is a clear candidate for medical treatment with indomethacin.

8. A 6-year-old boy is brought to the United States by his new adoptive parents from an orphanage in Eastern Europe. The boy is small for his age and has a bluish hue in the lips and tips of his fingers. He has clubbing and spells of cyanosis relieved with squatting. He has a systolic ejection murmur in the left third intercostal space. Chest x-ray shows a small heart and diminished pulmonary vascular markings. ECG shows right ventricular hypertrophy.

What is it? Tetralogy of Fallot. Cyanotic children could have any of the 5 conditions that begin with the letter "T":

- Tetralogy or transposition of the great vessels (common)
- Truncus arteriosus, total anomalous pulmonary venous connection, or tricuspid atresia (rare)

If the baby went home after birth, and later was found to be cyanotic, bet on tetralogy. If he was blue from the moment of birth, bet on transposition.

Management. Even if all you can recognize from the vignette is that the child has cyanosis, start with an echocardiogram as a good diagnostic test. The intricate details of surgical correction are bound to be beyond the level of knowledge expected on the exam.

ACQUIRED HEART DISEASE

1. A 72-year-old man has a history of angina and exertional syncopal episodes. He has a harsh midsystolic heart murmur best heard at the right second intercostal space and along the left sternal border.

What is it? Aortic stenosis with the triad of angina, dyspnea, and syncope.

Management. Diagnose with echocardiogram. Surgical valvular replacement is indicated if there is a gradient of >50 mm Hg, or at the first indication of CHF, angina, or syncope.

2. A 72-year-old man has been known for years to have a wide pulse pressure and a blowing, high-pitched, diastolic heart murmur best heard at the right second intercostal space and along the left lower sternal border with the patient in full expiration. He has had periodic echocardiograms, and in the most recent one there is evidence of beginning left ventricular dilatation.

What is it? Chronic aortic insufficiency.

Management. Aortic valve replacement.

3. A 26-year-old drug-addicted man develops CHF over a short period of a few days. He has a loud, diastolic murmur at the right, second intercostal space. A physical examination done a few weeks ago, when he had attempted to enroll in a detoxification program, was completely normal.

What is it? Acute aortic insufficiency caused by endocarditis.

Management. Emergency valve replacement, and antibiotics for a long time.

4. A 35-year-old woman has dyspnea on exertion, orthopnea, paroxysmal nocturnal dyspnea, cough, and hemoptysis. She has had these progressive symptoms for about 5 years. She looks thin and cachectic and has atrial fibrillation and a low-pitched, rumbling diastolic apical heart murmur. At age 15 she had rheumatic fever.

What is it? Mitral stenosis.

Management. Start with echocardiogram. Eventually, consider surgical mitral valve repair.

5. A 55-year-old woman has been known for years to have mitral valve prolapse. She now has developed exertional dyspnea, orthopnea, and atrial fibrillation. She has an apical, high-pitched, holosystolic heart murmur which radiates to the axilla and back.

What is it? Mitral regurgitation.

Management. Start with the echocardiogram. Eventually, consider surgical repair of the valve (annuloplasty) or valve replacement.

6. A 55-year-old man has progressive, unstable, disabling angina that does not respond to medical management. His father and 2 older brothers died of heart attacks age <50. The patient stopped smoking 20 years ago, but still has a sedentary lifestyle, is a bit overweight, has type 2 diabetes mellitus, and has high cholesterol.

What is it? It's a heart attack waiting to happen: this man needs a cardiac catheterization to see whether he is a suitable candidate for coronary revascularization.

7. A 55-year-old man has progressive, unstable, disabling angina that does not respond to medical management. His father and 2 older brothers died of heart attacks age <50. The patient stopped smoking 20 years ago, but still has a sedentary life style, is a bit overweight, has type 2 diabetes mellitus, and has high cholesterol. Cardiac catheterization demonstrates 70% occlusion of 3 coronary arteries, with good distal vessels. His left ventricular ejection fraction is 55%.

Management. The patient is lucky. He has good distal vessels (smokers and diabetics often do not) and enough cardiac function left. He clearly needs coronary bypass, and with triple-vessel disease he is not a good candidate for angioplasty.

8. A postoperative patient who underwent open heart surgery is determined to have a cardiac index 1.7 L/min/m^2 and left ventricular end-diastolic pressure 3 mm Hg.

The postoperative management of open heart surgery is too esoteric for the exam, but a bit of applied physiology is not. You should be able to recognize a dangerously low cardiac index, without a high end-diastolic pressure—a clear indication for increased fluid intake.

9. A 72-kg patient who had a triple coronary bypass is determined on postoperative day 2 to have a cardiac output of 2.3 L/min. Pulmonary wedge pressure is 27 mm Hg. Cardiac output is low, but the ventricle is failing.

Management. Cardiac output of 2.3L/min in a 72-kg patient is an indicator of heart failure. Given the elevated pulmonary wedge pressure, hypovolemia is not the issue. In the post-CABG period, myocardial dysfunction is common and inotropic support is indicated. Common pharmacological agents for this scenario include epinephrine, norepinephrine, and dobutamine.

LUNG

1. On a routine pre-employment physical examination, a chest x-ray is done on a 45-year-old chronic smoker. A solitary pulmonary nodule is found in the upper lobe of the right lung.

What is it? The concern, of course, is cancer of the lung.

Diagnosis. Find an older chest x-ray if one is available (from ≥1 year ago). The workup for cancer of the lung is expensive and invasive. On the other hand, cancer of the lung grows and kills in a predictable way, over a matter of several months. If an older x-ray has the same unchanged lesion, it is not likely cancer. No further workup is needed now, but the lesion should be followed with periodic x-rays.

2. A 65-year-old man with a 40 pack-year history of smoking gets a chest x-ray because of persistent cough. A peripheral, 2-cm solitary nodule is found in the right lung. A chest x-ray taken 2 years ago was normal.

3. A 66-year-old man with a 40 pack-year history of smoking gets a chest x-ray because of persistent cough. A peripheral 2-cm solitary pulmonary nodule is found in the right lung. A chest x-ray taken 2 years ago was normal. CT scan shows no calcifications in the mass, no liver metastases, and no enlarged peribronchial or peritracheal lymph nodes. Sputum cytology, bronchoscopy, and percutaneous needle biopsy have not been diagnostic. The man has good pulmonary function and is otherwise in good health.

Management. In dealing with cancer of the lung, 3 issues are at play:
- Establishing the diagnosis, which sometimes requires very invasive steps
- Ascertaining whether surgery can be done, i.e., will the patient still be functional after some lung tissue is removed
- Determining whether the surgery has a fair chance to cure him? (It will not if the tumor is extensive.)

Here is an example of a man who could stand lung resection (peripheral lesion, good function) and who stands a good chance for cure (no node metastases in the CT scan). Diagnostic steps should be VATS or wedge resection to remove the wedge of tissue one suspects for malignancy.

4. A 72-year-old chronic smoker with severe COPD is found to have a central, hilar mass on chest x-ray. Sputum cytology establishes a diagnosis of squamous cell carcinoma of the lung. His forced expiratory volume in 1 second (FEV1) is 1,100 ml, and a ventilation–perfusion scan shows that 60% of his pulmonary function comes from the affected lung.

Management. The history and physical exam suggested that the main limiting factor would be pulmonary function, so that issue was properly evaluated first. It takes an FEV1 of at least 800 ml to survive surgery and not be a pulmonary cripple afterward. If this patient underwent a pneumonectomy (which he would need for a central tumor), he would be left with FEV1 440 ml. No way. Don't do any more tests. He is not a surgical candidate. You already have a diagnosis to pursue chemotherapy and radiation.

5. A 62-year-old chronic smoker has an episode of hemoptysis. Chest x-ray shows a central hilar mass. Bronchoscopy and biopsy establish a diagnosis of squamous cell carcinoma of the lung. His FEV1 is 2,200 ml, and a ventilation–perfusion scan shows that 30% of his pulmonary function comes from the affected lung.

Management. This patient could tolerate a pneumonectomy, but we still have to determine the extent of his disease. CT scan alone may be able to establish that he does not have metastasis. CT plus PET scan may be required in some cases where the status of the mediastinal nodes is not clear, and if the PET scan cannot provide an answer, an endobronchial U/S to sample nodes would be the next step in management.

6. A 33-year-old woman undergoes a diagnostic workup because she appears to have Cushing syndrome. Chest x-ray shows a central 3-cm round mass on the right lung. Bronchoscopy and biopsy confirm a diagnosis of small cell carcinoma of the lung.

Management. Radiation and chemotherapy. Small cell lung cancer is not treated with surgery, and thus we have no need to determine FEV1 or nodal status.

1. A 54-year-old right handed laborer notices coldness and tingling in his left hand as well as pain in the forearm when he does strenuous work. What really concerned him, though, is that in the last few episodes he also experienced transitory vertigo, blurred vision, and difficulty articulating his speech.

This is subclavian steal syndrome. A combination of claudication of the arm with posterior brain neurologic symptoms is classic for this rare but fascinating (and thus favorite question) condition. Duplex scanning will demonstrate retrograde flow through the vertebral artery when the patient exercises the arm. Surgical bypass resolves the problem.

2. A 62-year-old man is found on physical examination to have a 6-cm pulsatile mass deep in the abdomen, between the xiphoid and the umbilicus.

This is an abdominal aortic aneurysm. He needs elective surgical repair, but because our decisions are based so much on the size of the aneurysm, we need more precise measurement. CT scan is indicated.

3. A 62-year-old man has vague, poorly described epigastric and upper back discomfort. He is found on physical examination to have a 6-cm pulsatile mass deep in the abdomen, between the xiphoid and the umbilicus. The mass is tender to palpation.

This is an abdominal aortic aneurysm that is beginning to leak. Get an immediate vascular surgery consultation as surgical repair is necessary.

4. A 68-year-old man is brought to the ED with excruciating back pain that began suddenly 45 minutes ago. He is diaphoretic and has a systolic BP 90 mm Hg. There is an 8-cm, pulsatile mass palpable deep in the abdomen, above the umbilicus.

The aneurysm is rupturing right now. He needs immediate, emergency surgery.

5. A wealthy, retired man has claudication when walking more than 15 blocks.

Vascular surgery and angioplastic stenting are palliative procedures; they do not cure arterio-sclerotic disease.

Claudication has an unpredictable course; thus, there is no indication for early operation or intervention. No expensive workup is needed. If he smokes, he should quit, and he would benefit from a program of exercise and the use of cilostazol.

6. A 56-year-old postman describes severe pain in his right calf when he walks 2 or 3 blocks. The pain is relieved by resting 10 or 15 minutes, but recurs if he walks again the same distance. He cannot do his job this way, and he does not qualify yet for retirement, so he is most anxious to have this problem resolved. He does not smoke.

This patient needs help. Start with Doppler studies. If he has a significant gradient, CT angio or MRI angio comes next, followed by bypass surgery or stenting.

7. A patient consults you because he "cannot sleep." On questioning it turns out that he has pain in the right calf, which keeps him from falling asleep. He relates that the pain goes away if he sits by the side of the bed and dangles the leg. His wife adds that she has watched him do that, and she has noticed that the leg, which was very pale when he was lying down, becomes deep purple several minutes after he is sitting up. On physical examination the skin of that leg is shiny, there is no hair, and there are no palpable peripheral pulses.

Rest pain. Definitely he needs the studies to see whether vascular surgery could help him.

8. A 45-year-old man shows up in the ED with a pale, cold, pulseless, paresthetic, painful, and paralytic lower extremity. The process began suddenly 2 hours ago. Physical examination shows no pulses anywhere in that lower extremity. Pulse at the wrist is 95/min, grossly irregular.

What is it? Embolization by the broken-off tail of a clot from the left atrium. Start with Doppler studies. If he has complete occlusion, do embolectomy with Fogarty catheters, and if he was ischemic for several hours, add a fasciotomy to prevent compartment syndrome. Incomplete occlusion may be treated with clot busters.

9. A 74-year-old man has sudden onset of extremely severe, tearing chest pain that radiates to the back and migrates down shortly after its onset. His BP is 220/110 mm Hg, and he has unequal pulses in the upper extremities and a wide mediastinum on chest x-ray. ECG and cardiac enzymes are negative for MI.

This is dissecting aneurysm of the thoracic aorta. Spiral CT scan is the best study to confirm the diagnosis in a noninvasive way. If the aneurysm is in the ascending aorta, emergency surgery should be performed. If it is in the descending aorta, intensive therapy in the ICU for the hypertension is the preferable option.

Skin Surgery 8

1. A 65-year-old West Texas farmer of Swedish ancestry has an indolent, raised, waxy, 1.2-cm skin mass over the bridge of the nose that has been slowly growing over the past 3 years. There are no enlarged lymph nodes in the head and neck.

2. A 71-year-old Arizona farmer of Irish ancestry has a non-healing, indolent, punched out, clean-looking 2-cm ulcer over the left temple that has been slowly becoming larger over the past 3 years. There are no enlarged lymph nodes in the head and neck.

Basal cell carcinoma has 2 potential configurations: waxy raised lesion or punched out ulcer, but both have a preference for the upper part of the face.

Diagnosis is made with full-thickness biopsy at the edge of the lesion (punch or knife) or complete excision with narrow margin of uninvolved skin. Management is surgical excision with clear margins, but conservative width. Alternatives include electrodessication with curettage or ablation.

3. A blond, blue-eyed, 69-year-old sailor has a non-healing, indolent 1.5-cm ulcer on the lower lip that has been slowly enlarging, for the past 8 months. He is a pipe smoker, and he has no other lesions or physical findings.

What is it? Squamous cell carcinoma. The location is classic.

Diagnosis. Biopsy, as described before.

Management. He will need surgical resection with wider (~1 cm) clear margins. Local radiation therapy is another option.

4. A red-headed, highly freckled, 23-year-old woman who worships the sun consults you for a concerning skin lesion on the shoulder. She has a pigmented lesion that is asymmetric, with irregular borders of different colors within the lesion. It measures 1.8 cm.

What is it? This is the classic ABCD which should alert you to melanoma or a forerunner (dysplastic nevus).

Management. Diagnosis made by excisional biopsy with a narrow margin is preferred. Once diagnosis is confirmed, definitive treatment is wide local excision with margins based on depth of invasion (Breslow). Sentinel lymph node biopsy is indicated for lesions >1 cm Breslow thickness.

5. A 35-year-old blond, blue-eyed man left his native Minnesota at age 18 and has been living an idyllic life as a crew member for a sailing yacht charter operation in the Caribbean. He has multiple nevi all over his body, but one of them has changed recently.

What is it? Change in a pigmented lesion is the other tip off to melanoma. It may be growth, or bleeding, or ulceration, or change in color—whatever. Manage as above.

6. A 44-year-old man has unequivocal signs of multiple liver metastases, but no primary tumor has been identified by multiple diagnostic studies of the abdomen and chest. The only abnormality in the physical examination is a missing toe, which he says was removed at age 18 for a black tumor under the toenail.

What is it? A classic vignette for malignant melanoma (the alternate version has a glass eye, and history of enucleation for a tumor). No self-respecting malignant tumor would have this time interval, but melanoma will.

7. A 32-year-old man had a 3.4-mm deep melanoma removed from the middle of his back 3 years ago. He now has… (a tumor in a weird place, like his left ventricle, his duodenum, his ischiorectal area–anywhere!).

The point of this vignette is that invasive melanoma (it has to be deep) metastasizes to all the usual places (lymph nodes plus liver-lung-brain-bone) but it is also the all-time-champion in going to weird places where few other tumors dare to go. Because tumor behavior is unpredictable in any given patient, doctors tend to be aggressive in resecting these metastases.

Ophthalmology 9

CHILDREN

1. A 1-year-old child is suspected of having strabismus. You verify that indeed the corneal reflection from a bright light in your examining room comes from different places from each of his eyes.

2. A 2-year-old child is diagnosed with a congenital cataract obstructing his vision in the right eye.

What is the point of these vignettes? To remind you that the brain "learns" to see what the eyes see during early infancy (up to about age 7). If one eye cannot see (any kind of obstruction) or the brain does not like what it sees (double vision), the brain will refuse to process the image and that cortical "blindness" will be permanent (the concept of amblyopia).

Management. The problem has to be surgically corrected as early as possible.

3. A young mother is visiting your office for routine medical care. She happens to have her 18-month-old baby with her, and you happen to notice that one of the pupils of the baby is white, whereas the other one is black.

What is it? An ophthalmologic and potentially life-and-death emergency. A white pupil (leukocoria) at this age can be retinoblastoma. This child needs to see the ophthalmologist not next week, but today or tomorrow. If it turns out to be something more innocent, like a cataract, it still needs correction to avoid amblyopia.

ADULTS

1. A 53-year-old woman arrives in the ED complaining of extremely severe frontal headache and nausea. The pain started about an hour ago, shortly after she left the movies where she watched a double feature. On further questioning, she reports seeing halos around the lights in the parking lot when she left the theater. On physical examination the pupils are mid-dilated and do not react to light. The corneas are cloudy with a greenish hue, and the eyes feel "hard as a rock."

What is it? A classic description of acute glaucoma. Not the most common type (most are asymptomatic—but you cannot write a vignette for those), but one that requires immediate treatment.

Management. An ophthalmologist is needed right away—but start treatment with systemic carbonic anhydrase inhibitors, topical beta-blockers, and alpha-2–selective adrenergic agonists. Mannitol and pilocarpine may also be used.

2. A 32-year-old woman presents in the ED with swollen, red, hot, tender eyelids on the left eye. She has fever and leukocytosis. When prying the eyelids open, you can ascertain that her pupil is dilated and fixed and that she has very limited motion of that left eye.

What is it? Orbital cellulitis.

Management. Another ophthalmologic emergency that requires immediate consultation, but if asked what to do, CT scan will be indicated to assess the extent of the orbital infection, and surgical drainage will follow.

3. A frantic mother reaches you on the phone, reporting that her 10-year-old boy accidentally splashed Drano (clogged drain remover) on his face. He is screaming in pain, complaining that his right eye hurts terribly.

Management. Copious irrigation is the main treatment for chemical burns. The point of this vignette is to remind you that time is a key element. If the mother is instructed to bring the boy to the ED, his eye will be cooked to a crisp by the time he arrives. The correct answer here is to instruct the mother to pry the eye open under cold water from the tap at home, and irrigate for 30 minutes before bringing the child to the hospital. You will do more irrigation in the ED, remove solid matter, and eventually recheck the pH before the child goes home. Do not forget to check the eyelid for remaining bits of Drano.

4. A 59-year-old, myopic gentleman reports "seeing flashes of light" at night when his eyes are closed. Further questioning reveals that he also sees "floaters" during the day, that they number 10 or 20, and that he also sees a cloud at the top of his visual field.

What is it? This is retinal detachment; 1–2 floaters would not mean that but >12 is an ominous sign. The "cloud" at the top of the visual field is hemorrhage settling at the bottom of the eye.

Management. Another ophthalmologic emergency. The retina specialist will use laser treatment to "spot weld" the retina and prevent further detachment.

5. A 77-year-old man suddenly loses sight from the right eye. He calls you on the phone 10 minutes after the onset of the problem. He reports no other neurologic symptoms.

What is it? Embolic occlusion of the retinal artery.

Management. Another ophthalmologic emergency—although little can be done for the problem, he has to get to the ED instantly. It might help for him to take an aspirin and breathe into a paper bag en route, and have someone press hard on his eye and release it repeatedly.

6. A 55-year-old man is diagnosed with type 2 diabetes mellitus. On questioning about eye symptoms, he reports that sometimes after a heavy dinner the television becomes blurry, and he has to squint to see it clearly.

What is it? The blurry TV is no big deal: the lens swells and shrinks in response to swings in blood sugar—the important point is that he needs to start getting regular ophthalmologic follow-up for retinal complications. It takes 10–20 years for these to develop, but type 2 diabetes may be present that long before it is diagnosed.

NECK MASSES

Congenital

1. A 15-year-old girl has a round, 1-cm cystic mass in the midline of her neck at the level of the hyoid bone. When the mass is palpated at the same time that the tongue is pulled, there seems to be a connection between the two. The mass has been present for at least 10 years, but only recently bothered the patient because it got infected.

What is it? Thyroglossal duct cyst.

Management. Sistrunk operation (removal of the mass and the track to the base of the tongue, along with the medial segment of the hyoid bone). Some people insist that the location of the normal thyroid must be ascertained first with radioisotope scanning.

2. An 18-year-old woman has a 4-cm, fluctuant round mass on the side of her neck, just beneath and in front of the sternocleidomastoid. She reports that it has been there at least 10 years, although she thinks that it has become somewhat larger in the last year or two. A CT scan shows the mass to be cystic.

This is a branchial cleft cyst. Do elective surgical removal.

3. A 6-year-old child has a mushy, fluid-filled mass at the base of the neck that has been noted for several years. The mass is ~6 cm in diameter, occupies most of the supraclavicular area and seems by physical examination to go deeper into the neck and chest.

What is it? Cystic hygroma.

Management. Get a CT scan to see how deep the mass goes. Cystic hygromas can extend down into the chest and mediastinum. Surgical removal will eventually be done.

Inflammatory versus Neoplastic

4. A 22-year-old woman notices an enlarged lymph node in her neck. The node is in the jugular chain, measures ~1.5 cm, is not tender, and was discovered by the patient yesterday. The rest of the history and physical examination are unremarkable.

Management. Before you spend a lot of money doing tests, let time be your ally. Schedule the patient to be rechecked in 3 weeks. If the node has gone away by then, it was inflammatory and nothing further is needed. If it's still there, it could be neoplastic and something needs to be done. Three weeks of delay will not significantly impact the overall course of a neoplastic process.

5. A 22-year-old woman seeks help regarding an enlarged lymph node in her neck. The node is in the jugular chain, measures ~2 cm, is firm, not tender, and was discovered by the patient 6 weeks ago. There is a history of low-grade fever and night sweats for the past 3 weeks. Physical examination reveals enlarged lymph nodes in both axillas and in the left groin.

What is it? Lymphoma.

Management. Tissue diagnosis will be needed. You can start with FNA of the available nodes, but eventually node biopsy will be needed to establish not only the diagnosis but also the type of lymphoma.

6. A 72-year-old man has a 4-cm hard mass in the left supraclavicular area. The mass is movable and not tender and has been present for 3 months. The patient has had a 20-pound weight loss in the past 2 months, but is otherwise asymptomatic.

What is it? Malignant metastases to a supraclavicular node from a primary tumor below the neck (Virchow's node). The vignette may include a few clues to suggest which one.

Diagnosis. Look for the obvious primary tumors: lung, stomach, colon, pancreas, kidney. The node itself may eventually be biopsied.

7. A 69-year-old man who smokes and drinks and has rotten teeth has a hard, fixed, 4-cm mass in his neck. The mass is just medial and in front of the sternocleidomastoid muscle, at the level of the upper notch of the thyroid cartilage. It has been there for at least 6 months, and it is growing.

What is it? Metastatic squamous cell carcinoma to a jugular chain node, from a primary in the mucosa of the head and neck (oropharyngeal–laryngeal territory).

Management. Don't biopsy the node! FNA is okay, but the best answer is triple endoscopy (examination under anesthesia of the mouth, pharynx, larynx, esophagus, and tracheobronchial tree), also known as a panendoscopy. CT scan will follow, to determine extent and operability. Most patients get combined therapy that includes radiation, platinum-based chemotherapy, and surgery if possible.

Squamous Cell Cancer—Other Presentations

8. A 69-year-old man who smokes and drinks and has rotten teeth has hoarseness that has persisted for 6 weeks in spite of antibiotic therapy.

9. A 69-year-old man who smokes and drinks and has rotten teeth has a painless ulcer in the floor of the mouth that has been present for 6 weeks and has not healed.

10. A 23-year-old man with AIDS has a painless ulcer in the floor of the mouth that has been present for 6 weeks and has not healed. He does not smoke or drink.

11. A 69-year-old man who smokes and drinks and has rotten teeth has a unilateral earache that has not gone away in 6 weeks. Physical examination shows serous otitis media on that side, but not on the other.

What are they? These are all different ways for squamous cell carcinoma of the mucosa of the head and neck to show up. They all need triple endoscopy to find and biopsy the primary tumor and to look for synchronous second primaries. Although the classic candidate for this disease is the older man who smokes and drinks, patients with AIDS also have very high incidence—with similar presentations.

OTHER TUMORS

1. A 52-year-old man complains of hearing loss. When tested he is found to have unilateral sensory hearing loss on one side only. He does not engage in any activity (such as sport shooting) that would subject that ear to noise that spares the other side.

What is it? Unilateral versions of common ENT problems in the adult suggest malignancy. In this case, acoustic nerve neuroma. Note that if the hearing loss had been conductive, a cerumen plug would be the obvious first diagnosis.

Diagnosis. MRI looking for the tumor.

2. A 56-year-old man develops slow, progressive paralysis of the facial nerve on one side. It took several weeks for the full-blown paralysis to become obvious, and it has been present now for 3 months. It affects both the forehead and the lower face.

What is it? Gradual, unilateral nerve paralysis suggests a neoplastic process.

Diagnosis. Gadolinium-enhanced MRI.

3. A 45-year-old man presents with a 2-cm firm mass in front of the left ear, which has been present for 4 months. The mass is deep to the skin, and it is painless. The patient has normal function of the facial nerve.

What is it? Pleomorphic adenoma (mixed tumor) of the parotid gland.

Diagnosis. FNA is appropriate, but the point of the question will be to bring out the fact that parotid masses are never biopsied in the office or under local anesthesia. Look for the option that offers referral to a head and neck surgeon for formal superficial parotidectomy which serves as a diagnostic and therapeutic tool.

4. A 65-year-old man presents with a 4-cm hard mass in front of the left ear, which has been present for 6 months. The mass is deep to the skin, and it is fixed. He has constant pain in the area, and for the past 2 months has had gradual progression of left facial nerve paralysis. He has rock-hard lymph nodes in the left neck.

This one is parotid cancer, but the point is the same: let the experts manage it.

PEDIATRIC ENT

1. A 2-year-old has unilateral earache.

2. A 2-year-old has unilateral foul-smelling purulent rhinorrhea.

3. A 2-year-old has unilateral wheezing, and the lung on that side looks darker on x-rays (more air) than the other side.

What is it? Unilateral versions of common bilateral ENT conditions in toddlers suggest foreign body (small toys). Appropriate x-rays, physical examination or endoscopies, and extraction are needed—obviously under anesthesia.

ENT EMERGENCIES AND MISCELLANEOUS

1. A 45-year-old woman with a history of a recent tooth infection shows up with a huge, hot, red, tender fluctuant mass occupying the left lower side of the face and upper neck, including the underside of the mouth. The mass pushes up the floor of the mouth on that side. She is febrile.

What is it? Ludwig's angina (an abscess of the floor of the mouth).

Management. The special issue is the need to maintain an airway. Incision and drainage are needed, but intubation or tracheostomy may also be required.

2. A 29-year-old woman calls your office at 10 AM with the history that she woke up that morning with one side of her face paralyzed.

Obviously Bell's palsy. The latest trend is to start these patients right away on antiviral medication and steroids.

3. A patient with multiple trauma from a car accident is being attended to in the ED. As multiple invasive things are done to him, he repeatedly grimaces with pain. The next day it is noted that he has a facial nerve paralysis on one side.

What is it? Trauma to the temporal bone can certainly transect the facial nerve, but when that happens the nerve is paralyzed right there and then. Paralysis appearing late is from edema. The point of the vignette is that nothing needs to be done.

4. Your office receives a phone call from Mrs. Rodriguez, a middle-aged patient whom you have treated repeatedly over the years for episodes of sinusitis. In fact, 6 days ago you started her on decongestants and oral antibiotics for what you diagnosed as frontal and ethmoid sinusitis. Now she tells you over the phone that ever since she woke up this morning, she has been seeing double.

What is it? Cavernous sinus thrombosis, or orbital cellulitis.

Management. This is a real emergency. She needs immediate hospitalization, high-dose IV antibiotic treatment, and surgical drainage of the paranasal sinuses or the orbit. CT scan will be needed to guide the surgery, but I expect that the thrust of the question will be directed at your recognition of the serious nature of this problem.

5. A 10-year-old girl has epistaxis. Her mother says that she often picks her nose.

What is it? Bleeding from the anterior part of the septum.

Management. Phenylephrine spray and local pressure.

6. An 18-year-old boy has epistaxis. The patient denies picking his nose. No source of anterior bleeding can be seen by physical examination.

What is it? In this age group either septal perforation from cocaine abuse, or posterior juvenile nasopharyngeal angiofibroma. The former may need posterior packing. The latter needs to be surgically removed (they are benign, but they eat away at nearby structures).

7. A 72-year-old, hypertensive man, on aspirin for arthritis, has a copious nosebleed. His BP is 220/115 mm Hg when seen in the ED. He says he began swallowing blood before it began to come out through the front of his nose.

What is it? Obviously epistaxis secondary to hypertension.

Management. These are serious problems that can end up with death. Medical treatment to lower the BP is clearly needed, and may be the option offered in the answers, but getting the ENT people there right away should also be part of the equation. Posterior packing is needed, emergency arterial ligation or angiographic embolization may be required.

8. A 57-year-old man seeks help for "dizziness." On further questioning he explains that he gets light-headed and unsteady, but the room is not spinning around.

What is it? Neurologic, probably vascular occlusive—but not inner ear. Direct your management and workup in that direction.

9. A 57-year-old man seeks help for "dizziness." On further questioning, he explains that the room spins around him.

What is it? This one is in the vestibular apparatus. I could not even begin to tell you how to work it up, but seek the answers that look like either symptomatic treatment (meclizine, Phenergan, diazepam) or an ENT workup.

VASCULAR OCCLUSIVE DISEASE

1. A 62-year-old right-handed man has transient episodes of weakness in the right hand, blurred vision, and difficulty expressing himself. There is no associated headache, the episodes have sudden onset, lasting about 5 or 10 minutes at the most, and they resolve spontaneously, leaving no neurologic sequela.

What is it? Transient ischemic attacks in the territory of the left carotid artery, caused by stenosis or an ulcerated plaque at the left carotid bifurcation.

Management. Start workup with Duplex scanning. If stenosis exceeds 70% proceed to carotid endarterectomy.

2. A 61-year-old man presents with a 1-year history of episodes of vertigo, diplopia, blurred vision, dysarthria, and instability of gait. The episodes have sudden onset, last several minutes, have no associated headache, and leave no neurologic sequela.

What is it? Another version of transient ischemic attacks, but now the vertebrals may be involved.

Management. Start with Duplex scanning.

3. Last week, a 60-year-old diabetic man had abrupt onset of right third nerve paralysis and contralateral hemiparesis. There was no associated headache. The patient is alert, but the neurologic deficits have not resolved.

What is it? Neurologic catastrophes that begin suddenly and have no associated headache are vascular occlusive. The vernacular for this man's problem is "a stroke."

Management. Vascular surgery in the neck is designed to prevent strokes, not to treat them once they happen. There are very rare exceptions, but revascularization of an ischemic brain area risks making it bleed and get worse. This patient will get a CT scan to assess the extent of the infarct and supportive treatment with emphasis on rehabilitation. Eventually his neck vessels will be looked at by Duplex to see whether a second stroke elsewhere may be preventable. If the vignette had given the patient a very early stroke, where IV infusion of tissue-type plasminogen activator (tPA) could be started within 90 minutes of the onset of symptoms, your choice would have been a CT scan (to rule out extensive or hemorrhagic infarcts), followed by the tPA infusion.

Intracranial Bleeding

4. A 64-year-old black man complains of a very severe headache of sudden onset and then lapses into a coma. Past medical history reveals untreated hypertension, and examination reveals a stuporous man with profound weakness in the left extremities.

What is it? Neurologic catastrophes of sudden onset, with severe headache, are vascular hemorrhagic. This man has bled into his head. In the vernacular, he has also suffered "a stroke."

Management. Give supportive measures with eventual rehabilitation efforts if he survives. CT scan is the universal first choice to see blood inside the head (we use it in trauma for the same purpose). This man will get one, to see exactly where he bled, and how bad it is.

5. A 39-year-old woman presents to the ED with a history of a severe headache of sudden onset that she says is different and worse than any headache she has ever had before. Her neurologic examination is completely normal, so she is given pain medication and sent home. She improves over the next few days, but 10 days after the initial visit she again gets a sudden, severe, and singular diffuse headache, and she returns to the ED. This time she has some nuchal rigidity on physical exam.

What is it? This one is a classic: subarachnoid bleeding from an intracranial aneurysm. The "sentinel bleed" that is not identified is a common feature. The "sudden, severe, and singular" nature of the pain is very common. And the nuchal rigidity betrays the presence of blood in the subarachnoid space.

Diagnosis. We are looking for blood inside the head, thus start with CT. Angiograms will eventually follow, in preparation for surgery to clip the aneurysm or endovascular coiling.

BRAIN TUMOR

1. A 31-year-old nursing student developed persistent headaches that began approximately 4 months ago, have been gradually increasing in intensity, and are worse in the mornings. For the past 3 weeks, she has been having projectile vomiting. Thinking that she may need new glasses, she seeks help from her optometrist, who discovers that she has bilateral papilledema.

What is it? Brain tumor. Neurologic processes that develop over a period of a few months and lead to increased ICP spell out tumor. Morning headaches are typical. If the tumor is in a "silent" area of the brain, there may be no other neurologic deficits.

Management. If given the option, pick MRI as your diagnostic test. If it is not offered, pick CT scan. Measures to decrease ICP while awaiting surgery include high-dose steroids (Decadron).

2. A 42-year-old right-handed man has a history of progressive speech difficulties and right hemiparesis for 5 months. He has had progressively severe headaches for the last 2 months. At the time of admission he is confused and vomiting and has blurred vision, papilledema, and diplopia. Shortly thereafter his BP goes up to 190 over 110, and he develops bradycardia.

What is it? Again brain tumor, but now with 2 added features: there are localizing signs (left hemisphere, parietal, and temporal area), and he manifests the Cushing reflex of extremely high ICP.

Management. As above, but as an emergency.

3. A 42-year-old man has been fired from his job because of inappropriate behavior. For the past 2 months he has gradually developed very severe, "explosive" headaches that are located on the right side, above the eye. Neurologic examination shows optic nerve atrophy on the right, papilledema on the left, and anosmia.

What is it? Brain tumor in the right frontal lobe. A little knowledge of neuroanatomy can help localize tumors. The frontal lobe has to do with behavior and social graces, and is near the optic nerve and the olfactory nerve. If you want the fancy name, this is the Foster Kennedy syndrome.

Management. MRI and neurosurgery.

4. A 12-year-old boy is short for his age, has bitemporal hemianopsia, and has a calcified lesion above the sella in x-rays of the head.

What is it? Craniopharyngioma.

Management. Get the fancy MRI and proceed with craniotomy.

5. A 23-year-old nun presents with a history of amenorrhea and galactorrhea of 6 months' duration. She is very concerned that others might think that she is pregnant, and she vehemently denies such a possibility.

What is it? Prolactinoma.

Management. First confirm that she indeed is not pregnant or hypothyroid. Then, since you suspect a functioning tumor of an endocrine gland, measure the appropriate hormone. So, here you want a prolactin level. You also want to see the tumor. The top choice for that is MRI. Bromocriptine therapy is favored by most, with surgery reserved for those who do not respond or who wish to become pregnant.

6. A 44-year-old man is referred for treatment of hypertension. His physical appearance is impressive: he has big, fat, sweaty hands, large jaw and thick lips, a large tongue, and huge feet. He is also found to have a touch of diabetes. In further questioning he admits to headaches, and he relates that his wedding ring no longer fits his finger.

What is it? Acromegaly. Appearance is so striking that the vignette is likely to come with a picture (or two: front including his hands, and lateral showing the large jaw).

Management. Somatomedin C determination, MRI, and eventually pituitary surgery or radiation therapy.

7. A 15-year-old girl has gained weight and become "ugly." She shows a picture of herself taken a year ago, where she was a lovely young woman. Now she has a hairy, red, round face full of pimples; her neck has a posterior hump, and her supraclavicular areas are round and convex. She has a fat trunk and thin extremities. She has mild diabetes and hypertension.

What is it? Cushing's syndrome. This one will also come with a picture, rather than a description. (Or two pictures, the before and after.)

Management. The sequence already described in the endocrine section: overnight low-dose dexamethasone suppression test. If no suppression, 24-hour urinary cortisol. If cortisol is high, do high-dose dexamethasone suppression test. If she suppresses at high dose, do an MRI of the sella, and follow with trans-sphenoidal pituitary surgery.

8. A 27-year-old woman develops a severe headache of sudden onset, making her stuporous. She is taken to the hospital, where she is found at admission to have a BP of 75 over 45. Funduscopic examination reveals bilateral pallor of the optic nerves. Relatives indicate that for the past 6 months, she has been complaining of morning headaches, loss of peripheral vision, and amenorrhea. After she developed the severe headache, and just before she went into a deep stupor, she told her relatives that her peripheral vision had suddenly deteriorated even more than before.

What is it? Pituitary apoplexy. (She has bled into a pituitary tumor.)

Management. Steroid replacement is urgently needed. Other hormones will need to be replaced eventually. MRI or CT scan will determine extent of the problem.

9. A 32-year-old man complains of progressive, severe generalized headaches that began 3 months ago, are worse in the mornings, and lately have been accompanied by projectile vomiting. He has lost his upper gaze, and he exhibits the physical finding known as "sunset eyes."

What is it? Another classic. This tumor is in the pineal gland, and if you want the fancy name, it is Parinaud syndrome.

Management. MRI to start. The neurosurgeons will take care of the rest.

10. A 6-year-old boy has been stumbling around the house and complaining of severe morning headaches for the past several months. While waiting in the office to be seen, he assumes the knee-chest position as he holds his head. Neurologic examination demonstrates truncal ataxia.

What is it? Tumor of the posterior fossa. Most brain tumors in children are located there, and cerebellar function is affected.

Management. MRI, neurosurgery.

11. A 23-year-old man develops severe headaches, seizures, and projectile vomiting over a period of 2 weeks. He has low-grade fever, and was recently treated for acute otitis media and mastoiditis.

What is it? Brain abscess. Signs and symptoms suggestive of brain tumor that develop in a couple of weeks with fever and an obvious source of infection spell out abscess.

Management. These are seen in CT as well as they would on MRI, and the CT is cheaper and easier to get…so pick CT if offered. Then the abscess has to be resected.

SPINAL CORD

1. A 52-year-old woman has constant, severe back pain for 2 weeks. While working in her yard, she suddenly falls and cannot get up again. When brought to the hospital she is paralyzed below the waist. Two years ago she had a mastectomy for cancer of the breast.

What is it? Most tumors affecting the spinal cord are metastatic, extradural. In this case the source is obvious, and the sudden onset of the paralysis suggests a fracture with cord compression or transection.

Management. Typically, an x-ray of the affected area is done right away, and it will show a huge, bony metastasis and the fracture that it has produced. But the best imaging to see what has happened to the cord (compressed? transected?) is the MRI. Neurosurgeons may be able to help if the cord is compressed rather than transected.

2. A 45-year-old man gives a history of aching back pain for several months. He has been told that he had muscle spasms, and was given analgesics and muscle relaxants. He comes in now because of the sudden onset of very severe back pain that came on when he tried to lift a heavy object. The pain is "like an electrical shock that shoots down his leg," it is worse with sneezing and straining, and it prevents him from ambulating. He keeps the affected leg flexed. Straight leg-raising test gives excruciating pain.

What is it? Lumbar disk herniation. Peak incidence is age 40s, and virtually all of these are at L4–L5 or L5–S1.

- If the "lightning" exits the foot by the big toe, it is L4–L5.
- If the "lightning" exits by the little toe, it is L5–S1.

Management. MRI for diagnosis. Bed rest and pain control will take care of most of these cases. Neurosurgical intervention is done only if there is progressive weakness or sphincteric deficits.

3. A 79-year-old man complains of leg pain brought about by walking and relieved by rest. On further questioning it is ascertained that he has to sit down or bend over for the pain to go away. Standing at rest will not do it. Furthermore, he can exercise for long periods of time if he is "hunched over," such as riding a bike or pushing a shopping cart. He has normal pulses in his legs.

What is it? The symptom is neurogenic claudication. The disease is spinal stenosis.

Management. Get MRI and refer to pain clinic. Pain control can usually be obtained with steroid and analgesic injections under x-ray guidance. Surgery is rarely needed for these.

4. A business executive who has been a T6 paraplegic for many years is held at a business meeting for several hours beyond the time when he would normally have done his in-and-out self-catheterization of the urinary bladder. He develops a pounding headache, profuse perspiration, and bradycardia. BP is 220/120 mm Hg.

The classic picture of autonomic dysreflexia. Obviously his bladder needs to be emptied, but he also needs alpha-adrenergic blocking agents and may benefit from calcium-channel blockers (such as nifedipine).

PAIN SYNDROMES

1. A 60-year-old man complains of extremely severe, sharp, shooting pain in his face, like a "bolt of lightning," that is brought about by touching a specific area and lasts about 60 seconds. His neurologic examination is normal, but it is noted that part of his face is unshaven because he fears to touch that area.

What is it? Tic douloureux (trigeminal neuralgia).

Management. Rule out organic lesions with MRI. Treat with anticonvulsants.

2. Several months after sustaining a crushing injury of his arm, a patient complains bitterly about constant, burning, agonizing pain that does not respond to the usual analgesic medications. The pain is aggravated by the slightest stimulation of the area. The arm is cold, cyanotic, and moist.

What is it? Causalgia (reflex sympathetic dystrophy).

Management. A successful sympathetic block is diagnostic, and surgical sympathectomy will be curative.

UROLOGIC EMERGENCIES

1. A 14-year-old boy presents in the ED with very severe pain of sudden onset in his right testicle. There is no fever, pyuria, or history of recent mumps. The testis is swollen, exquisitely painful, "high riding," and with a "horizontal lie." The cord is not tender.

What is it? Testicular torsion, a urologic emergency.

Management. Emergency surgery to save the testicle (bilateral orchiopexy). Do not waste time doing diagnostic studies.

2. A 24-year-old man presents in the ED with very severe pain of recent onset in his right scrotal contents. There is a fever of 103°F and pyuria. The testis is in the normal position, and it appears to be swollen and exquisitely painful. The cord is also very tender.

What is it? Acute epididymitis.

Management. This is the condition that presents the differential diagnosis with testicular torsion. Torsion is a surgical emergency epididymitis is not. This patient does not need to be rushed to the OR; all he needs is antibiotic therapy.

Should a diagnosis of testicular torsion be missed, the medicolegal implications are so severe that urologists routinely do a sonogram when they are sure the problem is epididymitis—just to absolutely, unequivocally rule out torsion.

3. A 72-year-old man is being observed with a ureteral stone that is expected to pass spontaneously. He develops chills, a temperature spike to 104°F, and flank pain.

What is it? Obstruction of the urinary tract alone is bad. Infection of the urinary tract alone is bad. But the combination of the two is horrible—a true urologic emergency. That's what this patient has.

Management. Massive IV antibiotic therapy, but the obstruction must also be relieved right now. In a septic patient, stone extraction would be hazardous, so the option in addition to antibiotics would be decompression by ureteral stent or percutaneous nephrostomy.

4. An adult woman relates that 5 days ago she began to notice frequent, painful urination, with small volumes of cloudy and malodorous urine. For the first 3 days she had no fever, but for the past 2 days she has been having chills, high fever, nausea, and vomiting. Also in the past 2 days she has had pain in the right flank. She has had no treatment whatsoever up to this time.

What is it? Pyelonephritis.

Management. UTI should not occur in men or in children, and thus should trigger a workup looking for a cause. Women of reproductive age, on the other hand, get cystitis all the time, and they are treated with appropriate antibiotics without great fuss. However, when they get flank pain and septic signs it's much more serious. This woman needs hospitalization, IV antibiotics, and at least a sonogram to make sure that there is no concomitant obstruction.

5. A 62-year-old man presents with chills, fever, dysuria, urinary frequency, diffuse low back pain, and an exquisitely tender prostate on rectal exam.

What is it? Acute bacterial prostatitis.

Management. This vignette is supposed to elicit from you what not to do. The treatment for this man is intuitive: he needs IV antibiotics—but what should not be done is any more rectal exams or any vigorous prostatic massage. Doing so could lead to septic shock.

6. A 33-year-old man has urgency, frequency, and burning pain with urination. The urine is cloudy and malodorous. He has mild fever. On physical examination the prostate is not warm, boggy, or tender.

The first part of this vignette sounds like prostatitis, which would be common and not particularly challenging; but if the prostate is normal on examination the ante is raised: The point of the vignette becomes that men (particularly young ones) are not supposed to get urinary tract infections. This infection needs to be treated, so ask for urinary cultures and start antibiotics—but also start a urologic workup. Do not start with cystoscopy (do not instrument an infected bladder, you could trigger septic shock). Start first with a sonogram.

CONGENITAL UROLOGIC DISEASE

1. You are called to the nursery to see an otherwise healthy-looking newborn boy because he has not urinated in the first 24 hours of life. Physical examination shows a big distended urinary bladder.

What is it? Infants are not born alive if they have no kidneys (without kidneys, lungs do not develop). This represents some kind of obstruction. First look at the meatus: it could be simple meatal stenosis. If it is not, posterior urethral valves is the best bet.

Management. Drain the bladder with a catheter if it passes easily (it will pass through the valves). Voiding cystourethrogram for diagnosis, endoscopic fulguration or resection for treatment.

2. A bunch of newborn boys are lined up in the nursery for you to do circumcisions. You notice that one of them has the urethral opening in the ventral side of the penis, about midway down the shaft.

What is it? Hypospadias.

The point of the vignette is that you don't do the circumcision. The foreskin may be needed later for reconstruction when the hypospadias is surgically corrected.

3. A newborn baby boy has one of his testicles down in the scrotum, but the other one is not. On physical examination the missing testicle is palpable in the groin. It can easily be pulled down to its normal location without tension, but it will not stay there; it goes back up.

What is it? This is a retractile testicle, due to an overactive cremasteric reflex.

Management. Nothing needs to be done now. Even truly undescended testicles may spontaneously descend during the first year of life. Those that do not require orchidopexy.

4. A 9-year-old boy gives a history of 3 days of burning on urination, with frequency, low abdominal and perineal pain, left flank pain, and fever and chills.

What is it? Little boys are not supposed to get UTI. There is more than meets the eye here. A congenital anomaly has to be ruled out.

Management. Treat the infection of course, but do IVP and voiding cystogram looking for reflux. If found, long-term antibiotics while the child "grows out of the problem."

5. A mother brings her 6-year-old girl to you because "she has failed miserably to get proper toilet training." On questioning you find out that the little girl perceives normally the sensation of having to void and voids normally and at appropriate intervals, but also happens to be wet with urine all the time.

What is it? A classic vignette: low implantation of one ureter. In little boys there would be no symptoms, because low implantation in boys is still above the sphincter, but in little girls the low ureter empties into the vagina and has no sphincter. The other ureter is normally implanted and accounts for her normal voiding pattern.

Management. If the vignette did not include physical exam, that would be the next step, which might show the abnormal ureteral opening. Often physical examination does not reveal the anomaly, and imaging studies would be required (start with IVP). Surgery will follow.

6.   A 16-year-old boy goes on a beer-drinking binge for the first time in his life. Shortly thereafter he develops colicky flank pain.

What is it? Another classic. Ureteropelvic junction obstruction.

Management. Start with U/S (sonogram). Repair will follow.

TUMORS

1.   A 62-year-old man reports an episode of gross, painless hematuria. Further questioning determines that the patient has total hematuria rather than initial or terminal hematuria.

What is it? The blood is coming anywhere from the kidneys to the bladder, rather than the prostate or the urethra. Either infection or tumor can produce hematuria. In older patients without signs of infection, cancer is the main concern, and it could be either renal cell carcinoma or transitional cell cancer of the bladder or ureter.

Management. Do a CT scan and cytoscopy.

2.   A 70-year-old man is referred for evaluation because of a triad of hematuria, flank pain, and a flank mass. He also has hypercalcemia, erythrocytosis, and elevated liver enzymes.

What is it? Full-blown picture of renal cell carcinoma (very rarely seen nowadays).

Management. Do a CT scan.

3.   A 55-year-old chronic smoker reports 3 instances in the past 2 weeks when he has had painless, gross, total hematuria. In the past 2 months he has been treated twice for irritative voiding symptoms, but has not been febrile, and urinary cultures have been negative.

What is it? Most likely bladder cancer but a renal etiology must be excluded.

Management. Do a CT scan and cytoscopy.

4.   A 59-year-old black man has a rock-hard, discrete, 1.5-cm nodule felt in his prostate during a routine physical examination.

5.   A 59-year-old black man is told by his primary care physician that his prostatic specific antigen (PSA) has gone up significantly since his last visit. He has no palpable abnormalities in his prostate by rectal exam.

What is it? The two classic presentations for early cancer of the prostate.

Management. Transrectal needle biopsy, guided by the examining finger in the first case, and guided by sonogram in the second. Eventually surgical resection or radiotherapy after the extent of the disease has been established.

6. A 62-year-old man had a radical prostatectomy for cancer of the prostate 3 years ago. He now presents with widespread bony pain. Bone scans show metastases throughout the entire skeleton, including several that are very large and very impressive.

Management. Significant, often dramatic palliation can be obtained with orchiectomy, although it will not be long-lasting (1 or 2 years only). An expensive alternative is luteinizing hormone-releasing hormone agonists, and another option is antiandrogens (flutamide).

7. A 78-year-old man comes in for a routine medical checkup. He is asymptomatic. When a physician had seen him 5 years earlier, a PSA had been ordered, but he notices as he leaves the office this time that the study has not been requested. He asks if he should get it.

Management. For many years PSA was not done after age 75. Improved longevity and better treatments for early prostatic cancer have led to a more flexible approach. Also, with the advent of robotic prostatectomy, the surgery is so much safer and with better outcomes that PSA is now being offered selectively.

8. A 25-year-old man presents with a painless, hard testicular mass. It is clear in the physical examination that the mass arises from the testicle rather than the epididymus. To be sure, a sonogram was done. The mass was indeed testicular.

What is it? Testicular cancer.

Management. This will sound horrible, but here is a disease where we shoot to kill first—and ask questions later. The diagnosis is made by performing a radical orchiectomy by the inguinal route. That irreversible, drastic step is justified because testicular tumors are almost never benign.

Beware of the option to do a trans-scrotal biopsy: that is a definite no-no. Further treatment will include lymph node dissection in some cases (too complicated a decision for you to know about) and platinum-based chemotherapy. Serum markers are useful for follow-up: α-fetoprotein and β-human chorionic gonadotropin (β-HCG), and they have to be drawn **before** the orchiectomy (but they do not determine the need for the diagnostic orchiectomy—that still needs to be done).

9.   A 25-year-old man is found on a pre-employment chest x-ray to have what appears to be a pulmonary metastasis from an unknown primary tumor. Subsequent physical examination discloses a hard testicular mass, and the patient indicates that for the past 6 months he has been losing weight for no obvious reason.

What is it? Same situation as earlier vignette, but with metastasis. The point of this vignette is that testicular cancer responds so well to chemotherapy that treatment is undertaken regardless of the extent of the disease when first diagnosed. Manage exactly as the previous case.

RETENTION AND INCONTINENCE

1.   A 60-year-old man shows up in the ED because he has not been able to void for the past 12 hours. He wants to, but cannot. On physical examination his bladder is palpable halfway up between the pubis and the umbilicus, and he has a big, boggy prostate gland without nodules. He gives a history that for several years now he has been getting up 4 or 5 times a night to urinate. Because of a cold, 2 days ago he began taking antihistaminics, using "nasal drops," and drinking plenty of fluids.

What is it? Acute urinary retention, with underlying benign prostatic hypertrophy.

Management. Indwelling bladder catheter, to be left in for at least 3 days. Further management will be based on the use of alpha-blockers. Other options include 5-alpha-reductase inhibitors for large glands, or newly developed noninvasive interventions. The traditional TURP is rarely done now.

2.   On postoperative day 2 after surgery for repair of bilateral inguinal hernias, a patient reports that he "cannot hold his urine." Further questioning reveals that every few minutes he urinates a few milliliters of urine. On physical examination there is a large palpable mass arising from the pelvis and reaching almost to the umbilicus.

What is it? Acute urinary retention with overflow incontinence.

Management. Indwelling bladder catheter.

3.   A 42-year-old woman consults you for urinary incontinence. She is the mother of 5 children. Ever since the birth of her last child 7 years ago, she leaks a small amount of urine whenever she sneezes, laughs, gets out of a chair, or lifts any heavy objects. She relates that she can hold her urine all through the night without any leaking whatsoever.

What is it? Stress incontinence.

Management. If she has no physical findings, she can be taught exercises that strengthen the pelvic floor. If she has a large cystocele, she will need surgical reconstruction.

STONES

1. A 72-year-old man who in previous years has passed 3 urinary stones is now again having symptoms of ureteral colic. He has relatively mild pain which began 6 hours ago but does not have much nausea and vomiting. CT scan shows a 3-mm ureteral stone just proximal to the ureterovesical junction.

Management. Urologists have a huge number of options to treat stones, including laser beams, shock waves, ultrasonic probes, baskets for extraction—but there is still a role for "watching and waiting." This man is a good example; it is a small stone, almost at the bladder. Give him time, medication for pain, and plenty of fluids, and he will probably pass it.

2. A 54-year-old woman has a severe ureteral colic. CT scan shows a 7-mm ureteral stone at the ureteropelvic junction.

Management. Whereas a 3-mm stone has a 70% chance of passing, a 7-mm stone only has a 5% probability of doing so. This one will have to be smashed and retrieved. The best option among choices offered would be shock-wave lithotripsy (SWL). (Contraindications to SWL include pregnancy, bleeding diathesis, and stones that are several centimeters big.)

MISCELLANEOUS

1. A 72-year-old man has for the past several days noticed bubbles of air coming out with the urine when he urinates. He also gives symptoms suggestive of mild cystitis.

What is it? Pneumaturia caused by a fistula between the bowel and the bladder. Most commonly from sigmoid colon to dome of the bladder, caused by diverticulitis. Cancer (also originating in the sigmoid) is the second possibility.

Management. Intuitively you would think that either cystoscopy or sigmoidoscopy would verify the diagnosis, but real life does not work that way: those seldom show anything. Contrast studies (cystogram or barium enema) are also typically unrewarding. The test to do is CT scan. Because ruling out cancer of the sigmoid is important, the sigmoidoscopic examination would be done at some point, but not as the first test. Eventually surgery will be needed.

2. A 32-year-old man has sudden onset of impotence. One month ago he was unexpectedly unable to perform with his wife after an evening of heavy eating and heavier drinking. Ever since then he has not been able to achieve an erection when attempting to have intercourse with his wife, but he still gets nocturnal erections and can masturbate normally.

What is it? Classic psychogenic impotence: young man, sudden onset, partner-specific.

Management. Curable with psychotherapy if promptly done.

3. Ever since he had a motorcycle accident where he crushed his perineum, a young man has been impotent.

4. Ever since he had an abdominoperineal resection for cancer of the rectum, a 52-year-old man has been impotent.

Organic impotence has sudden onset only when it is related to trauma. Vascular injury explains the first of these two, and vascular reconstruction may help. Nerve injury accounts for the second, and only prosthetic devices can help there.

5. A 66-year-old diabetic man with generalized arteriosclerotic occlusive disease notices gradual loss of erectile function. At first he could get erections, but they did not last long; later the quality of the erection was poor; and eventually he developed complete impotence. He does not get nocturnal erections.

This is the classic pattern of organic impotence (not related to trauma). A wide range of therapeutic options exists, but probably the first choice now is sildenafil, tadalafil, and vardenafil.

1. A 62-year-old man who had a motorcycle accident has been in a coma for several weeks. He is on a respirator, has had pneumonia on and off, has been on vasopressors, and shows no signs of neurologic improvement. The family inquires about brain death and possible organ donation.

At one time the medical profession was very fussy about who was accepted as an organ donor. Nowadays, with 65,000 patients on transplant waiting lists and many dying every day for lack of organs, almost anybody is taken. The rule now is that all potential donors are referred to the local organ harvesting organization. Donors with specific infections (such as hepatitis) can be used for recipients with the same infection. Even donors with metastatic cancer are eligible for eye donation.

A positive HIV status remains the only absolute contraindication to a patient serving as an organ donor.

2. Ten days after liver transplantation, levels of g-glutamyltransferase (GGT), alkaline phosphatase, and bilirubin begin to go up. There is no U/S evidence of biliary obstruction or Doppler evidence of vascular thrombosis.

3. On week 3 after a closely matched renal transplant, there are early clinical and laboratory signs of decreased renal function.

4. Two weeks after a lung transplant, the patient develops fever, dyspnea, hypoxemia, decreased FEV1, and interstitial infiltrate on chest x-ray.

There are 3 kinds of rejection. **Hyperacute rejection** happens within minutes of re-establishing blood supply, produces thrombosis, and is caused by preformed antibodies. ABO matching and lymphocytotoxic crossmatch prevent it, and thus we do not see it clinically—and you will not encounter it on the exam.

Acute rejection is the one we deal with all the time. It occurs after the first 5 days, and usually within the first few months. Signs of organ dysfunction (as in these vignettes) suggest it, but biopsy is what confirms it. In the case of the heart, there are no early clinical signs; thus biopsies there are done routinely at set intervals. Once diagnosed, the first line of therapy is steroid boluses. If unsuccessful, antilymphocyte agents are used (anti-thymocyte serum).

5. Several years after a successful (renal, hepatic, cardiac, pulmonary) transplantation, there is gradual, insidious loss of organ function.

The third form, **chronic rejection**, is poorly understood and irreversible. There is no treatment for it, but the correct answer for such vignette would be to do biopsy. Late acute rejection episodes could be the problem, and those can be treated.

Index

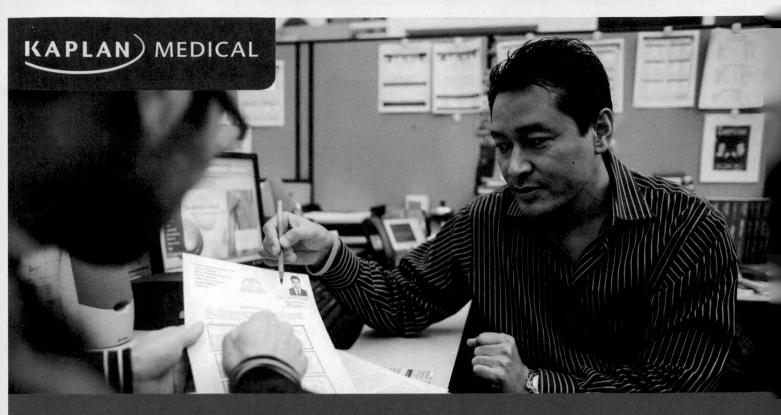

Improve your odds of matching.

Meet your medical advisor: your personal coach to USMLE® and the Match™.

Behind each champion, you will find a great coach. Schedule a complimentary 30-minute session with a medical advisor and connect with them via Skype, on the phone or in person.

You'll discuss your:
- personalized study plan
- Qbank and NBME® performance
- exam readiness
- residency application timeline

Our medical advisors know every exam and every part of the medical residency application process. They will help you understand every step you'll take on the road to residency.

Don't delay. Request your free med advising appointment today.

Visit **kaplanmedical.com/freeadvising**

USMLE® is a joint program of The Federation of State Medical Boards of the United States, Inc. and the National Board of Medical Examiners.